Bioinformatics Tools for Detection and Clinical Interpretation of Genomic Variations

Edited by Ali Samadikuchaksaraei and Morteza Seifi

Published in London, United Kingdom

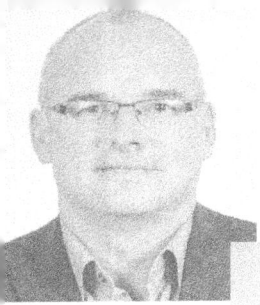
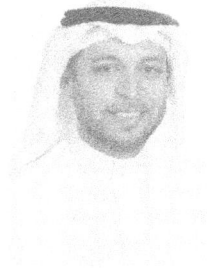
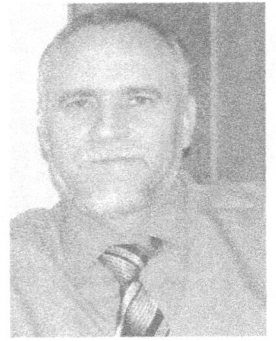
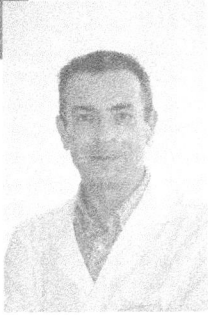
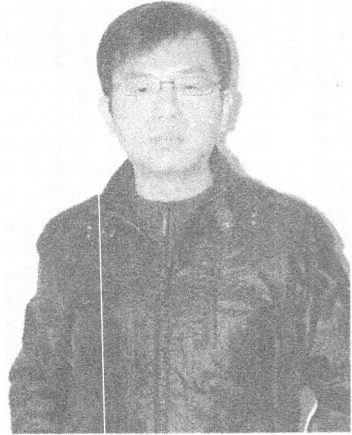
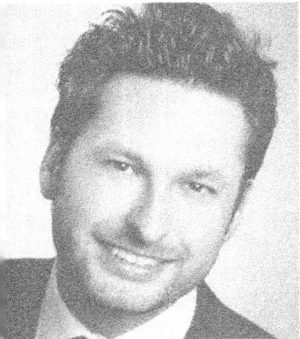
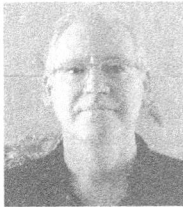

IntechOpen

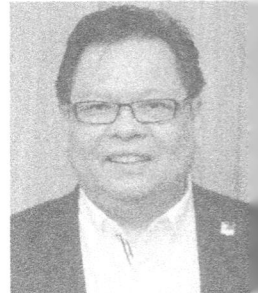
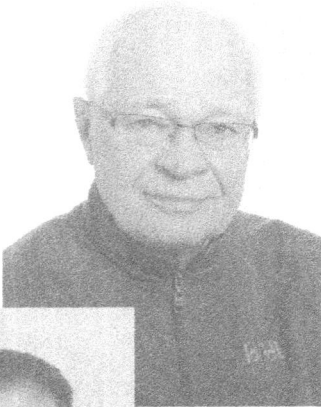
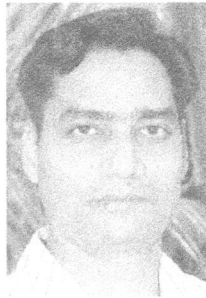
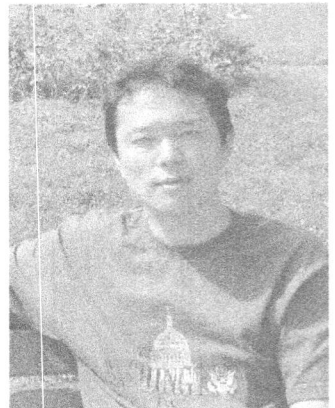
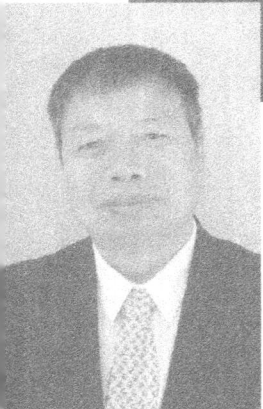
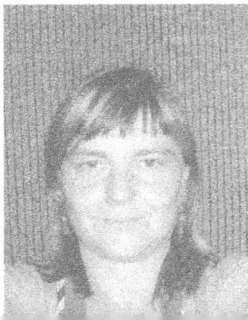

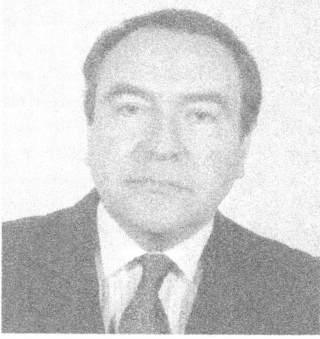

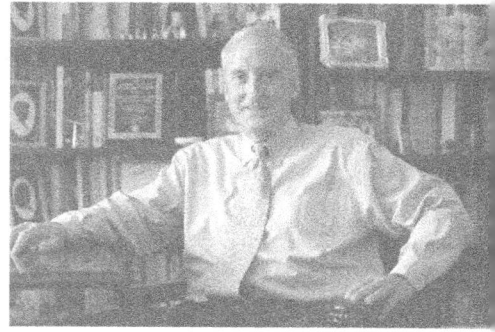

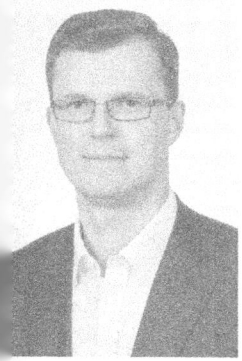

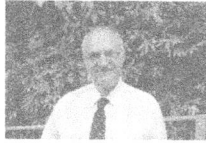

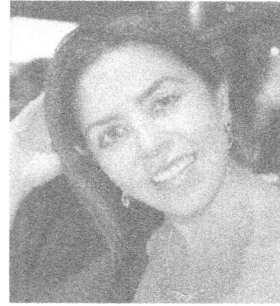

Supporting open minds since 2005

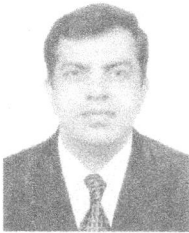

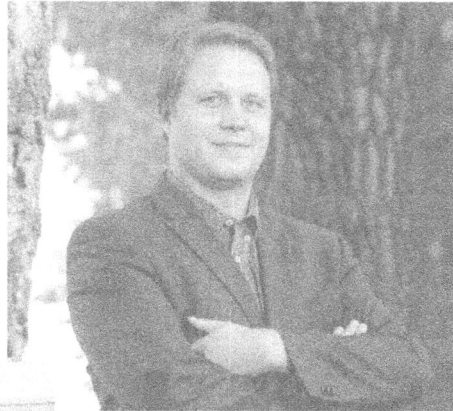

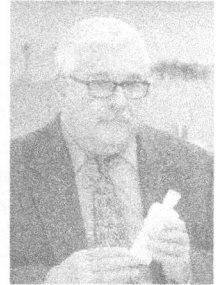

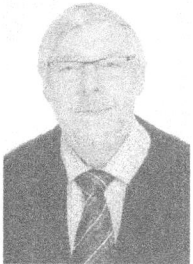

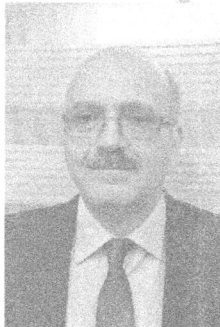

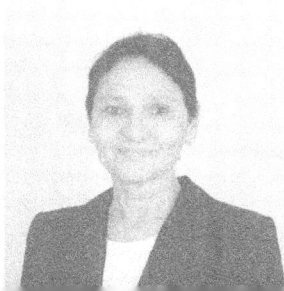

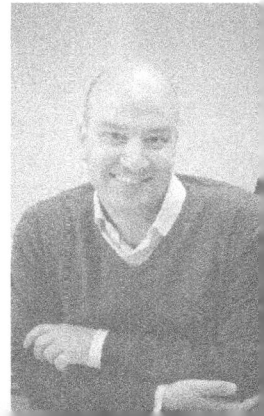

Bioinformatics Tools for Detection and Clinical Interpretation of Genomic Variations
http://dx.doi.org/10.5772/intechopen.77443
Edited by Ali Samadikuchaksaraei and Morteza Seifi

Contributors
Xianquan Zhan, Tian Zhou, Tingting Cheng, Miaolong Lu, Gaston K. Mazandu, Emile R. Chimusa, Ephifania Geza, Milaine Seuneu, Juliano Lino Ferreira, Leila Ferreira, Thelma Sáfadi, Tesfahun Alemu Setotaw, Osman Ugur Sezerman, Kok-Siong Poon, Evelyn Siew-Chuan Koay, Julian Wei-Tze Tang

Notice
Statements and opinions expressed in the chapters are these of the individual contributors and not necessarily those of the editors or publisher. No responsibility is accepted for the accuracy of information contained in the published chapters. The publisher assumes no responsibility for any damage or injury to persons or property arising out of the use of any materials, instructions, methods or ideas contained in the book.

First published in London, United Kingdom, 2019 by IntechOpen
IntechOpen is the global imprint of INTECHOPEN LIMITED, registered in England and Wales, registration number: 11086078, The Shard, 25th floor, 32 London Bridge Street
London, SE19SG - United Kingdom
Printed in Croatia

British Library Cataloguing-in-Publication Data
A catalogue record for this book is available from the British Library

Additional hard and PDF copies can be obtained from orders@intechopen.com

Bioinformatics Tools for Detection and Clinical Interpretation of Genomic Variations
Edited by Ali Samadikuchaksaraei and Morteza Seifi
p. cm.
Print ISBN 978-1-78923-799-3
Online ISBN 978-1-78923-800-6
eBook (PDF) ISBN 978-1-83881-844-9

We are IntechOpen,
the world's leading publisher of
Open Access books
Built by scientists, for scientists

4,200+

Open access books available

116,000+

International authors and editors

125M+

Downloads

151

Countries delivered to

Our authors are among the

Top 1%

most cited scientists

12.2%

Contributors from top 500 universities

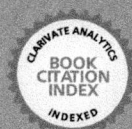

Interested in publishing with us?
Contact book.department@intechopen.com

Numbers displayed above are based on latest data collected.
For more information visit www.intechopen.com

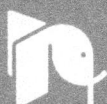

Meet the editors

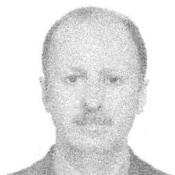

Ali Samadikuchaksaraei is a Professor of Medical Biotechnology, Tissue Engineering and Regenerative Medicine at Iran University of Medical Sciences. He is an expert in detection, analysis, and interpretation of clinically relevant genomic variations. As a well-known figure in this field, he is regularly consulted by the Iranian Academies, scientific organizations, and industrial sectors.

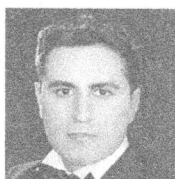

Dr. Morteza Seifi completed his PhD and postdoctoral training at the University of Alberta. He employs molecular and cellular techniques and bioinformatics tools to provide functional evidence of pathogenicity of genomic variations. Dr. Seifi has received several scholarships, awards, and grants, including one of Canada's largest and most prestigious endowments for academic activities, the Izaak Walton Killam Memorial Scholarship.

Contents

Preface

Genomic variations are the basis for phenotypic variations of individual organisms of the same species. These phenotypic variations could be of clinical importance in humans and medically relevant organisms. Therefore detection of genomic variations, and interpretation of their phenotypic effects and pathogenic potentials, has become a growing field in both biomedical research and clinical medicine.

Bioinformatics Tools for Detection and Clinical Interpretation of Genomic Variations is an up-to-date compilation of chapters on application of data analysis and mining tools for identification of clinically important genomic variations.

Chapter 1 discusses the application of non-decimated wavelet transform (NDWT) coupled with elastic net domains and Hurst exponent in identification of genetic diversity. Chapter 2 describes a comprehensive workflow for analysis of whole exome and whole genome sequencing data. It also presents the steps needed for variant discovery workflow with a particular focus on germline short variants and germline short insertion and deletion events. Additionally, this chapter outlines methods for analysis of somatic and structural variations.

Chapter 3 discusses local ancestry deconvolution and dating admixture events and the possible gaps in the knowledge that lead to the current challenges. Chapter 4 addresses the value of multiomics-based molecular patterns and the concept of pattern recognition and pattern biomarkers in cancer diagnosis and prognosis. It also explores the application of these concepts in personalized medicine. Chapter 5 addresses the genetic diversity of the hepatitis C virus and discusses its genotyping and concurrent variant profiling, as identification of resistance-associated variants of this virus determines the choice of anti-viral regimes in infected patients.

We would like to thank all the authors for their contributions and time in preparing this valuable collection. Also, we would like to extend our thanks to Mr. Luka Cvjetković for his great help during the editing of this book and to IntechOpen for their commitment and support.

Ali Samadikuchaksaraei, MD, PhD
Departments of Medical Biotechnology and Tissue Engineering
& Regenerative Medicine,
Iran University of Medical Sciences,
Tehran, Iran

Morteza Seifi, PhD
Alberta Children's Research Institute (ACRI),
Calgary, Alberta,
Canada

The Bioinformatics Tools for Discovery of Genetic Diversity by Means of Elastic Net and Hurst Exponent

Leila Maria Ferreira, Thelma Sáfadi,
Tesfahun Alemu Setotaw and Juliano Lino Ferreira

Abstract

The genome era allowed us to evaluate different aspects on genetic variation, with a precise manner followed by a valuable tip to guide the improvement of knowledge and direct to upgrade to human life. In order to scrutinize these treasured resources, some bioinformatics tools permit us a deep exploration of these data. Among them, we show the importance of the discrete non-decimated wavelet transform (NDWT). The wavelets have a better ability to capture hidden components of biological data and an efficient link between biological systems and the mathematical objects used to describe them. The decomposition of signals/sequences at different levels of resolution allows obtaining distinct characteristics in each level. The analysis using technique of wavelets has been growing increasingly in the study of genomes. One of the great advantages associated to this method corresponds to the computational gain, that is, the analyses are processed almost in real time. The applicability is in several areas of science, such as physics, mathematics, engineering, and genetics, among others. In this context, we believe that using R software and applied NDWT coupled with elastic net domains and Hurst exponent will be of valuable guideline to researchers of genetics in the investigation of the genetic variability.

Keywords: wavelet, genome, NDWT, elastic net, Hurst exponent

1. Introduction

The genome era allowed us to evaluate different aspects on genetic variation, with a precise manner followed with a valuable tip to guide the improvement of knowledge and direct to upgrade to human life. In order to scrutinize these treasured resources, some bioinformatics tools permit us a deep exploration of these data. Among them, we display the significance of the discrete non-decimated wavelet transform (NDWT). The wavelets they possess improved capability to identify occult constituents of biological data and do a well-organized connection amid biological systems and the mathematical items used to designate them. The decomposition of signals/sequences at diverse stages of resolution allows obtaining different characteristics in each level. The analysis using technique of wavelets has been growing increasingly in the study of genomes. One of the great advantages associated to this method corresponds to the computational gain, that is, the analyses are processed almost in real time. The applicability is in numerous themes of science, as physics, mathematics, engineering, genetics, meteorology, and oceanography, among others. The wavelet transform comprehends a technique of see and represents a signal. This signal is decomposed in resolution intensities, where each level brings a detailing. Mathematically, it is embodied by a function oscillating in time or space. As characteristic, it has sliding windows that expand or compress to capture low- and high-frequency signals. Its starting point arose in the field of seismic training to designate the instabilities ascending from a seismic impulse. Among the wavelets techniques, we have the discrete non-decimated wavelet transform (NDWT), whose main characteristic is that it can work with any size of signals/sequences. In this procedure, the inductance is paraphrase invariants, to be exact; the selection of origin is irrelevant, provided all the observations are used in the analysis, a condition that does not happen in the discrete decimated wavelet transform (DWT). The technique of discrete wavelet transforms is being used to find gene locations in genomic sequences, detecting long-range correlations, discovering periodicities in sequences of DNA and analysis of G + C patterns. The NDWT technique may be applied in any genome type, increasing the promptness of the analysis, because the analyses with this method are processed almost in real time. The wavelets have demonstrated to be an efficient method in the analysis of DNA sequences. This tool is imperative to be applied to elastic net. The main feature of the elastic net technique is the grouping of correlated variables where the quantity of predictors is greater than the quantity of remarks. Furthermore, the Hurst exponent allows the evaluation of genome similarities. In the same way, the NDWT is crucial to evaluate the Hurst exponent. Strictly speaking, the bioinformatics tool NDWT is a fundamental step to allow the examination of genomic variation through the other subsequent bioinformatics tools, like elastic net and Hurst exponent, which allow us to understand, interpret, and identify the genome variation in a certain species.

2. Wavelet

Wavelet analysis, nowadays, is used widely in subjects such as signal processing, engineering, physics, genetics, mathematics, medical sciences, economics, astronomy, etc. The genetic approach of this tool appears to be a valuable and interesting possibility in science.

Wavelet is miniature wave. Whatsoever their form has a distinct number of oscillations and lasts through a definite period of time or space. Wavelets hold countless appropriate properties. Wavelets possess gender categories: there are father wavelets φ and mother wavelets ψ. The father wavelet fits to 1, and the mother wavelet fits to 0. Wavelets also arise in different shapes. There are the discrete ones, the symmetric, the nearly symmetric, and the asymmetric. The key aspect of wavelet investigation is that it allows the researcher to separate out a variable or signal into its essential multiresolution components [1].

In the last 21 years, more than 2000 articles were published with wavelet technique in wide-ranging subjects.

Wavelet theory delivers an integrated background for number methods which had been established autonomously for several signal processing applications [2]. Wavelet concept is established on Fourier analysis [3], in which all function may be denoted as the sum of sine and cosine functions.

Non-decimal wavelet transform (NDWT) possesses ample spectra of application, including mammographic imaginings, geology, genomes, applied mathematics, applied physics, atmospheric sciences, and economics, among other applications. In our specific case, we will approach the genomic approach.

When working with the complete genome, which is all the heritable information of an organism that is set in DNA or, in some viruses, in RNA, this includes both the genes and the noncoding sequences of a specific species; the main feature we find is the large volume of data. To elucidate this problem, the technique called wavelets has emerged as an efficient alternative in data compression, owning one of the main advantages that this technique offers. However, wavelet functions are also commanding apparatuses in signal processing, noise elimination, separation of components in the signal, identification of singularities, and detection of self-similarity, among others.

The goals of this examination address to show how wavelets possibly will be used in the analysis of genome clustering using the energy and interaction of wavelet functions with data grouping techniques (elastic net and Hurst exponent).

Structure of the analysis: first it is required to acquire the signal of the genome that will be analyzed; for this purpose, it is used to the tool called GC content. The signal if is required to apply a wavelet transform, in this case the NDWT will be used, working with the Daubechies wavelet with a certain number of null moments. The amount of decomposition levels will depend on the size of the genome. The scalogram is calculated using the detail coefficients obtained through the decomposition levels. The clustering analysis is done using the dendrogram with medium binding and applying the Mahalanobis distance.

In order to apply the elastic net technique in wavelet transform (NDWT), all levels of decomposition are used; as a characteristic of this interaction, it is possible to see the groupings at each of the decomposition levels.

Applying the Hurst exponent technique on the levels of signal decomposition, each level brings information regarding the amount degree of Hurst exponent index. All values found for the Hurst exponent are used in the dendrogram with the mean binding and the distance of Mahalanobis. There are several methods of estimation of Hurst exponent; the most commonly used is the R/S method.

3. Wavelet transform

Wavelet analysis has arisen as a possible device for spectral investigation owing to the interval incidence localization which makes it appropriate for multifaceted and motionless signals. The wavelet transform has added meaningfully in the training of many processes/signals in virtually all areas of earth science [4].

Wavelet is mathematical function. To be considered a wavelet, it must have the total area on the function curve equals to zero. The energy of the behavior must be limited (regularity and well located). Another need in the art is the speed and ease of calculating the wavelet transform and the inverse transform.

Among various application areas of wavelets are computer vision, data compression, fingerprint compression at the FBI, data recovery affected by noise, similar behavior detection, musical tones, astronomy, meteorology, numerical image processing, and many others.

The wavelet transform rots a function demarcated in the period domain into another function, well-defined in time domain and frequency domain. It is defined as

$$W(a,b) = \int_{\infty}^{\infty} f(t) \frac{1}{\sqrt{|a|}} \psi^* \left(\frac{t-b}{a} \right) dt, \tag{1}$$

which is a behavior function of two real parameters, a and b. If we define $\psi_{a,b}(t)$ as

$$\psi_{a,b}(t) = \frac{1}{\sqrt{|a|}} \psi^* \left(\frac{t-b}{a} \right), \tag{2}$$

we may put another way the transform as the inner output of the functions $f(t)$ and $\psi_{a,b}(t)$:

$$W(a,b) = \langle f(t), \psi_{a,b}(t) \rangle = \int_{-\infty}^{\infty} f(t) \, \psi_{a,b}^*(t) dt. \tag{3}$$

The function $\psi(t)$ which equals $\psi_{1,0}(t)$ is entitled the mother wavelet, while the other functions $\psi_{a,b}(t)$ stay called daughter wavelets. The parameter b designates that the function $\psi(t)$ has been translated on the t axis of a distance equivalent to b, being then a translation parameter. The parameter causes a change of scale, increasing (if $a > 1$) or decreasing (if $a < 1$) the wavelet formed by the function. Consequently, the parameter "a" remains known as the scaling parameter.

4. Wavelet analysis

There are abundant types of wavelet transform. Rely on the procedure one can be desired that others. The wavelet analysis is prepared by the successive procedure of wavelet transform with several values for the criterion a and b, representing the decomposition of the signal components located in period and the agreeing to these parameters. Each wavelet has a better or worse location in the domains of frequency and of the time, so the analysis can be done with wavelets according to the desired result. Wavelet analysis brings with it an analysis of where the resolution level is set by the index a.

Discrete wavelets: among them are the Daubechies wavelet, wavelet of Cohen-Daubechies-Feauveau (occasionally mentioned as CDF N/P or Daubechies bior-thogonal wavelets), Beylkin [5], BNC wavelets, Coiflet, Mathieu wavelet, Haar wavelet, binomial-QMF, Villasenor wavelet, Legendre wavelet, and symlet.

Continuous wavelets: (1) the real-valued wavelets are Mexican hat wavelet, Hermitian wavelet, beta wavelet, Hermitian hat wavelet, and Shannon wavelet, and the (2) complex-valued wavelets are Shannon wavelet, Morlet wavelet, complex Mexican hat wavelet, and modified Morlet wavelet.

In the latest decades, the investigation using method of wavelets has been rising progressively. One of the great rewards related with this method links to the compu-tational improvement, that is, the analyses are treated virtually in real time. The applicability is in numerous areas of science, like physics, mathematics, engineer-ing, and genetics, among others.

The wavelet transform is a method of sighted and characterizes a signal. Mathematically, it is characterized by a function wavering in time or space. As a characteristic, it has sliding windows that increase or bandage to capture low- and high-frequency signals, respectively [2]. Its origin arose in the field of seismic study to define the instabilities ascending from a seismic impulse [6].

Among the wavelet techniques, we have the discrete non-decimated wavelet transform (NDWT), whose main characteristic is that it may work with any extent of signals/sequences.

In this procedure, the coefficients are translation invariants, that is, the selec-tion of source is unrelated since all the annotations are done in the investigation, a condition that does not happen in the discrete decimated wavelet transform (DWT).

In recent period, the discrete wavelet transforms were worn to find gene sites in sequences of the genome [7], finding long-range correlations, finding periodicities in sequences of the DNA molecule [8], and also in the scrutiny of G + C patterns [9].

The clustering analysis is often assumed to deal with DNA sequences proficiently. A wavelet-based element vector model was anticipated for grouping of DNA sequences [10].

The distinction of the discrete NDWT is to retain the similar extent of data in even and odd decimations on each measure and remain to do the identical on each subsequent scale, being D0 the dyadic decimation, D1 the odd decimation, H the high-pass filter, and L the low-pass filter. Consider, for example, an input path $(y_1, ..., y_n)$. Then, put on and preserve both $D_0 H_y$ and $D_1 H_y$, even and odd indexed of the observation-filtered wavelets. Each of these sequences is length $n/2$. Consequently, in whole, the amount of wavelet coefficients in both decimals on the better scale is $2 \times n/2 = n$ [11].

5. GC content

An important parameter in genetics is the GC content. They are referred as the percentage of each bases of nitrogen composition of the molecule of DNA or RNA. We own the adenine, cytosine, guanine, thymine, and uracil. They are called by the acronyms A, C, G, T, and U, respectively. The last one belongs to RNA molecule replacing thymine. They are applied to the complete genome or determined fragment. This concept may be applied in coding or noncoding molecule segment. The adenine has the same quantity of thymine (DNA) or uracil (RNA). The cytosine has the same sum of guanine in either RNA or DNA. The amount of GC is related to high-stability one which value is less than AT or AU. In the opposite is low stability when this quantity is relatively small compared with AT or AU. This detail is because GC has three hydrogen bonds, although AU or AT has two of them.

The GC proportion inside a genome is established to be evidently variable. The DNA coding section is straight proportional to stand-up G + G.

In varied organisms, GC content is found to be too variable, which donate the dissimilarities in recombination pattern, including association with DNA repair, selection, and in the alteration of mutational bias patterns. Due to the essence of the genetic coding, it is nearly incredible for an organism to have a genome with a GC content pending either 0 or 100%. An organism species with an exceptionally low GC content is *Plasmodium falciparum* having about 20% of GC amount, published at NCBI—available at https://www.ncbi.nlm.nih.gov/bioproject?cmd=Retrieve&dopt=Overview&list_uids=148.

The GC percentage is the largely used systematic approaches in many prokaryotic organisms mainly in bacteria species. Actinobacteria are one example of uppermost GC bacterial content. Another example is *Streptomyces coelicolor* being 72% of G + G amount.

Interestingly, the software apparatuses GCSpeciesSorter [12] and TopSort [13] are used for categorizing species centered on their GC contents.

6. Daubechies wavelet

The Daubechies wavelets, established on the study done by Ingrid Daubechies, comprise of a series of orthogonal wavelets determining a discrete wavelet transform and categorized by a greatest amount of disappearing moments for certain given provision. With every wavelet assembly of this category lies in a scaling function (entitled the father wavelet) that produces an orthogonal multiresolution investigation.

Ingrid Daubechies is a Belgian physicist and mathematician. Daubechies was the first female to be chair of the International Mathematical Union (2011–2014). She is very well acknowledged for her study using wavelets in image compression.

Daubechies earned the Louis Empain Prize for Physics in 1984, conferred once every 5 years to a Belgian scientist on the basis of a study done before the age of 29. In the middle of 1992 and 1997, she stood a partner of the MacArthur Foundation, in addition in 1993, she was designated to the American Academy of Arts and Sciences. In 1994, she earned the American Mathematical Society Steele Prize for explanation for her book *Ten Lectures on Wavelets* and was requested to provide an entire talk in Zurich at the International Congress of Mathematicians. In 1997, she stood granted the AMS Ruth Lyttle Satter Prize available at http://www.ams.org/profession/prizes-awards/pabrowse#year=1997. In 1998, she was selected to the United States National Academy of Sciences, which can be visualized at http://nas.nasonline.org/site/Dir/1753239219?pg=vprof&mbr=1001102&returl=http%3A%2F%2Fwww.nasonline.org%2Fsite%2FDir%2F1753239219%3Fpg%3Dsrch%26view%3Dbasic&retmk=search_again_link and acquired the Golden Jubilee Award for Technological Innovation from the IEEE Information Theory Society (https://www.itsoc.org/honors/golden-jubilee-awards-for-technological-innovation). She turns into an overseas fellow of the Royal Netherlands Academy of Arts and Sciences in 1999 accessible at https://www.knaw.nl/en/members/foreign-members/4013.

In 2000, Daubechies turns out to be the pioneer lady to obtain the National Academy of Sciences Award in Mathematics, stated every 4 years for excellence in published mathematical investigation. The prize honored her for important findings on wavelets and wavelet growths and designed for her accomplishment in building wavelet methods a constructive elementary apparatus of applied mathematics. This achievement is presented on https://www.knaw.nl/en/members/foreign-members/4013. She was also conferred the Basic Research Award, German Eduard Rhein Foundation, which could be visualized on https://web.archive.org/web/20110718233021/http://www.eduard-rhein-stiftung.de/html/Preistraeger_e.html and https://web.archive.org/web/20110718234059/http://www.eduard-rhein-stiftung.de/html/2000/G00_e.html and the NAS Prize in Mathematics https://web.archive.org/web/20101229195210/http://www.nasonline.org/site/PageServer?pagename=AWARDS_mathematics.

Generally, the Daubechies wavelet properties stay preferred to have the maximum sum A of vanishing moments (this does not make sure of indicating the preeminent levelness) on behalf of assumed provision measurement 2A-1 [3]. It is present in two designation patterns in routine, DN via the extent or total of blows and dbA stating to the quantity of vanishing moments. Thus db2 and D4 stand the equivalent wavelet transform.

Among the 2A-1 thinkable resolution of the arithmetical calculations for the moment and orthogonal circumstances, the one is elected whose scaling filter has extreme phase. Wavelet transform remains too easy to place hooked on training through the debauched wavelet transform. Daubechies wavelets are broadly used in answering wide-ranging problems, for example, self-homology assets of sign or fractal difficulties and sign cutoffs, among others.

Daubechies wavelets remain not demarcated in footings of the subsequent scaling and wavelet functions; actually, they are not probable to inscribe down in locked procedure.

In the production of a wavelet scaling arrangement, low-pass filter and the wavelet sequence band-pass filter will standardized to ensure entirety unenliven 2 and summation of squares unenliven 2. In particular requests, they are standardized to require sum√2; thus one and other arrangements and entirely changes of them by an even sum of coefficients are orthonormal to each other.

The employment of Daubechies wavelets though software such as Mathematica rope straight mode is available at https://reference.wolfram.com/language/ref/DaubechiesWavelet.html, a basic execution is humble in MATLAB. This application routines periodization to grip the problematic of limited measurement signals. Other, further refined devices are accessible, but habitually it is not required to use these as it merely touches the many split ends of the converted signal. The periodization is fulfilled in the onward transform straight in MATLAB vector system and the inverse transform by means of the circshift() function.

7. Non-decimal wavelet transform

Non-decimal wavelet transform (NDWT) has the benefits of period invariance and redundancy, paralleled to the typical orthogonal wavelet transformations. NDWT owns properties beneficial in various wavelet applications. Furthermore, NDWT matrix is capable to powerfully map a signal arising from an acquirement field to the wavelet sphere with humble matrix multiplication and deprived of the prerequisite of the whole quantity of the signal [14].

A widespread version of wavelet transform is a NDWT, which can overwhelm sensitivity to translations in time and change found in typical [15] orthogonal wavelet transform. Initially in the 1990s, NDWT arose in scientific literature using several names for a figure of applications and purposes [16].

A process that approaches nonstop wavelet transform with an iterative algorithm, which evicted to be corresponding to a shift-invariant representation, was put forward by [17]. Furthermore, a resourceful algorithm was defined with $O(n \log 2 (n))$ complexity for scheming wavelet coefficients that stand shift-invariant, to be exact, humble repetitious wavelet coefficients at wholly N circulant shift for an input signal size of N [5, 18]. In addition, a wavelet packet decomposition for time invariance and applied it to estimation and detection problems was proposed by Pesquet and collaborators [19] and lengthy finished in the study [20], uses an over ample wavelet decomposition, which is stated to as discrete wavelet frame, for arrangement of texture. After that, two other studies [21, 22] tested translation-invariant transform to verge for noise reduction. Then, the study of stationary wavelet transform with example applications for local spectra estimation was published [23]. Finally, an examination of applied translation-invariant wavelet algorithm for data compression was done [24].

The time-invariance property of NDWT generates a reduced mean square error and also reduces the Gibbs phenomenon in d-noising applications [21]. Conversely, the defilement of variance maintenance in NDWT embarrasses the signal restoration [16].

Major benefits of a NDWT matrix are squeezability, calculation promptness, and tractability in magnitude of an input signal. We previously deliberated the superior compressibility when NDWT matrices are well-worn for 2-D scale-mixing transforms.

NDWT possess ample spectra of application, including mammographic imaginings, geology, genomes, physics, atmospheric sciences, and economics, among other applications.

8. Scalogram

Spectrogram is an ample prevalent tool in signal analysis because it provides a scattering of signal energy in time-frequency plane. The wavelet spectrogram is broadly known like scalogram [25]. Comprehend a distribution of energy in timescale plane. The scalogram yields a more or less simply intelligible visual in two-dimensional representations of signals [26].

The scalogram is a valuable device for the understanding of the wavelet signal represented. It is like a graph of the square sum of the wavelet coefficients in different levels. In the occurrence of discrete transformation, it embodies a decomposition of function energy without timescale. One of its features is the aptitude to detect periodic components of the signal; either apparatuses will result in peaks in the scalogram. These apparatuses may be mined from the signal by dividing the ripple coefficients into different sets, where each of these sets is at the same peak. High- and low-frequency apparatuses of a signal might be restored by applying a reverse loop transformation to separate sets [27].

The energy $E\ (j)$ aimed at the wavelet d coefficients in each level j, which corresponds to the scalogram, is represented by

$$E(j) = \sum_{k=0}^{n} d_{j,k}^2 \quad para \quad j = 1, ..., J \tag{4}$$

9. Cluster analysis

Cluster analysis also known as unsupervised classification is a grouping of items into diverse groups, each of which requisite be assembled rendering to the rules of programming. This assembly must be handled computationally, without user intervention.

The term clustering analysis, early termed by [15], actually contains an assortment of different grouping algorithms, all of which address an important issue in several areas of research: how to organize observed data into structures that make sense or how to develop taxonomies capable of classifying data observed in different classes. Important is to even consider that these assembly must be classes that occur naturally in the dataset.

Clustering analysis is the designation given to the group of computational techniques whose purpose is to separate objects into groups, based on the characteristics that these objects have. The basic idea is to put objects in the same group that are similar in some predetermined criteria. The criterion is usually based on a dissimilarity function, which function receives two objects and returns the distance between them. The groups determined by a quality metric should have high internal and high homogeneity separation (external heterogeneity). This implies that the elements of a given set should be mutually similar and, preferably, have a high amount of differences from the elements of other sets [28].

Biologists, for instance, have to organize data observed in structures that make sense, that is, develop taxonomies. Microbiologists confronted with a variety range of species of a certain type, for example, must be capable to classify the observed specimens into clusters before it has been possible to describe these microorganisms in detail in ways to detach in detail the differences between species and subspecies.

Grouping procedures have been practiced in a huge range of areas. Ref. [29] already provides a broad overview of several published studies on the use of grouping analysis techniques. In the medical field, for example, grouping of diseases by symptom or cures can lead to very useful taxonomies. In areas of psychiatry, for example, clustering of syndrome, for instance, paranoia, schizophrenia, and others, is considered essential for proper therapy. In archeology, conversely, one has also tried to group civilizations or times of civilizations based on tools of stone, funerary objects, etc. In general, whenever a "mountain" of unknown data is required to be classified into manageable cells, grouping methods are used.

10. Elastic net

In statistics and specifically in the suitable of linear or logistic regression models, the elastic net is a standardized regression method that linearly couples the L1 and L2 punishments of the lasso and ridge approaches. **Figure 1** shows the elastic net typical design.

Lasso is a regression method broadly worn in domains with huge datasets, such as genomic data, where proficient and agile algorithms are vital [30]. Ridge regression is a procedure for investigating manifold regression data that arise out of multicollinearity. When multicollinearity arises, least squares estimates are unbiased, but their variances are huge so they might be outlying from the accurate value. In 1970, the investigation of [31] published an article about ridge regression, approaching the tendentious appraisal for nonorthogonal issues. In 2009, [32] study examined the ridge regression and their extensions applied to genome-wide selection into *Zea mays* L.

R software, available at https://www.r-project.org/, has the packing necessary to do a wavelet and elastic net based on genome sequence. Furthermore, the elastic net may be also used with microsatellite (SSR) data. This tool could be used in any genetic data of all organisms.

The most relevant article about elastic net was published in 2005 [33]. They say that elastic net is of pronounced interest especially when the predictors' number is considerably higher than the sum of observations. This might be useful in real or in simulation data.

The recent evolution of science brought a fast deeper understanding of the genome. In this sense, through several methods with varying levels of complexity added to the computational efficiency at the present days, we may easily compare organisms based on their genetic dissimilarity. Along these lines, we used accurate

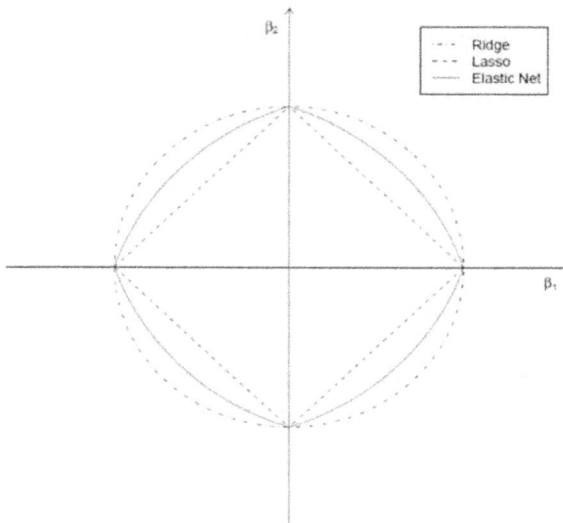

Figure 1.
Elastic net standard scheme.

genomic selection methods dropping the penalties of each approaches like in elastic net, enabling the fitting of a certain statistical model. Therefore, an outstanding methodology to analyze genome is elastic net domain used in several study, like [33–36].

Recently, the tuberculosis strain's differences were evaluated using the elastic net domain [34]. In that examination, 10 genome sequences of *Mycobacterium tuberculosis* with a window size of 10,000 bp were assessed combining the NDWT and elastic net domain. This study encompasses 10 strains: 2 from drug resistant, 6 from drug susceptible, 1 from multidrug resistant, and finally 1 from extensively drug resistant. The clustering detected on that analysis indicated to be real adequate.

11. Hurst exponent

Hurst exponent is applied as a degree of long-standing memory of time series. It associates to the autocorrelations of time series and the degree at which these decline as the lag between pairs of values intensifications. This coefficient has started to be established in hydrology, used to understand the variation level of dam size at Nile River over a long cycle of time. Harold Edwin Hurst was a British engineer that worked with hydrology; for this reason the coefficient has his surname. Later, this exponent was used in several areas, including fractal geometry, storage process, trends in financial market analyzing economic time series, mechanics, physics, mathematics, computation, and finally to the long-ranging dependency in DNA. **Figure 2** displays the values of Hurst exponent and their interpretation in a long-standing.

Using the genetic data, the Hurst exponent approach is able to build genetic cluster based on genome sequence. There are a lot of estimation methods of Hurst exponent: the original and best-known is the alleged rescaled range (R/S) analysis promoted by [37, 38] and based on previous hydrological findings [39]. Alternatives include DFA, periodogram regression [40] aggregated variances [41], local Whittle's estimator [42], and wavelet analysis [43, 44] both in the time domain and frequency domain.

In our case, we performed a Hurst exponent in the bacterial strains used in article [34]. We did many methods of Hurst exponent. Interestingly, the R/S methodology was the most similar to the cluster obtained on elastic net domain approach. This data is not shown due to being in a review process to an International journal currently. Our data agree with the majority of scientific papers published approaching the Hurst exponent, which so far applying the R/S method.

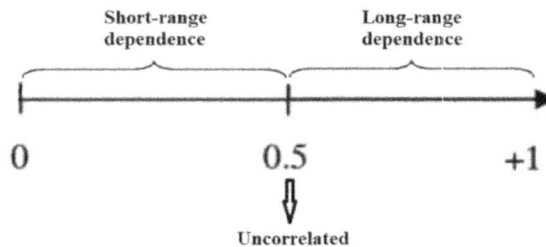

Figure 2.
Hurst exponent pattern interpretation of the index value.

12. Conclusion

We strongly believe that exploring the genetic variability of any organism using wavelet coupled with elastic net domain and/or Hurst exponent will be a valuable and interesting tool. It is not difficult and the free R software could solve easily the approach. In this way, it gives reliability and robustness in your results. Therefore, these bioinformatics apparatuses provide more possibility to scrutinize the genetic divergence of living organisms.

Conflict of interest

The authors do not have conflict of interests.

Author details

Leila Maria Ferreira[1], Thelma Sáfadi[1], Tesfahun Alemu Setotaw[2] and Juliano Lino Ferreira[3*]

1 Universidade Federal de Lavras, Lavras, Minas Gerais, Brazil

2 Ethiopian Institute of Agricultural Research, Addis Ababa, Ethiopia

3 Empresa Brasileira de Pesquisa Agropecuária, Bagé, Rio Grande do Sul, Brazil

*Address all correspondence to: juliano.ferreira@embrapa.br

IntechOpen

References

[1] Crowley PM. A guide to wavelets for economists. Journal of Economic Surveys. 2007;**21**:207-267. DOI: 10.1111/j.1467-6419.2006.00502.x

[2] Percival DB, Walden AT. Wavelet Methods for Time Series. 1st ed. Cambridge: Analysis Cambridge University Press; 2000. 594 p. DOI: 10.1017/CBO9780511841040

[3] Dodin G, Vandergheynst P, Levoir P, et al. Fourier and wavelet transform analysis, a tool for visualizing regular patterns in DNA sequences. Journal of Theoretical Biology. 2000;**206**:323-326

[4] Chamoli A. Wavelet analysis of geophysical time series. e-Journal Earth Science India. 2009;**2**:258-275

[5] Beylkin G. On the representation of operators in bases of compactly supported wavelets. SIAM Journal on Numerical Analysis. 1992;**29**:1716-1740

[6] Morlet J, Arens G, Fourgeau E, Giard D. Wave propagation and sampling theory–Part II: Sampling theory and complex waves. Geophysics. 1982;**47**:222-236. DOI: 10.1190/1.1441329

[7] Ning J, Moore CN, Nelson JC. Preliminary wavelet analysis of genomic sequences. In: Proceedings of the IEEE Computer Society Conference on Bioinformatics CSB '03. Stanford, California: IEEE; 2003. pp. 509-510

[8] Vannucci M, Liò P. Non-decimated wavelet analysis of biological sequences: Applications to protein structure and genomics. Sankhyā: The Indian Journal of Statistics, Series B. 2001;**63**:218-233. DOI: 10.2307/25053172

[9] Daubechies I. Ten Lectures on Wavelets. 1st ed. Berlin: Springer-Verlag; 1992. 344 p

[10] Bao J, Yuan RY. A wavelet-based feature vector model for DNA clustering. Genetics and Molecular Research. 2015;**14**:19163-19172. DOI: 10.4238/2015.December.29.26

[11] Nason G. Wavelet Methods in Statistics with R. 1st ed. New York: Springer-Verlag; 2008. 259 p. DOI: 10.1007/978-0-387-75961-6

[12] Karimi K, Wuitchik D, Oldach M, Vize P. Distinguishing species using GC contents in mixed DNA or RNA sequences. Evolutionary Bioinformatics Online. 2018;**14**:1-4. DOI: 10.1177/1176934318788866

[13] Lehnert E, Mouchka M, Burriesci M, Gallo N, Schwarz J, Pringle J. Extensive differences in gene expression between symbiotic and aposymbiotic cnidarians G3: Genes, genomes. Genetics. 2014;**4**: 277-295. DOI: 10.1534/g3.113.009084

[14] Zhou H, Narayanan RM. Microwave imaging of non-sparse object using dual-mesh method and iterative method with adaptive thresholding. IEEE Transactions on Antennas and Propagation. 2018; early access. DOI: 10.1109/TAP.2018.2876164

[15] Tryon RC. Cluster Analysis: Correlation Profile and Orthometric (Factor) Analysis for the Isolation of Unities in Mind and Personality. 1st ed. Ann Arbor: Edwards Brothers; 1939. 122 p

[16] Kang M. Non-decimated wavelet transform in statistical assessment of scaling: Theory and applications [thesis]. Atlanta: Georgia Institute of Technology; 2016

[17] Mallat S. Zero-crossings of a wavelet transform. IEEE Transactions on Information Theory. 1991;**37**:1019-1033. DOI: 10.1109/18.86995

[18] Shensa MJ. The discrete wavelet transform: Wedding the a trous and mallat algorithms. IEEE Transactions on Signal Processing. 1992;**40**:2464-2482. DOI: 10.1109/78.157290

[19] Pesquet JC, Krim H, Carfantan H. Time-invariant orthonormal wavelet representations. IEEE Transactions on Signal Processing. 1996;**44**:1964-1970

[20] Unser M. Texture classification and segmentation using wavelet frames. IEEE Transactions on Image Processing. 1995;**4**:1549-1560

[21] Coifman RR, Donoho DL. Translation-invariant de-noising. In: Antoniadis A, Oppenheim G, editors. Wavelets and Statistics. Lecture Notes in Statistics. Vol. 103. New York: Springer; 1995. pp. 1-26. DOI: 10.1007/978-1-4612-2544-7_9

[22] Lang M, Guo H, Odegard JE, Burrus CS, Wells RO Jr. Nonlinear processing of a shift-invariant discrete wavelet transform (dwt) for noise reduction. In: Szu HH, editor. Wavelet Applications. 2nd ed. Orlando: Proc. SPIE 2491; 1995. pp. 640-651. DOI: 10.1.1.24.4098

[23] Nason GP, Silverman BW. The stationary wavelet transform and some statistical applications. In: Antoniadis A, Oppenheim G, editors. Wavelets and Statistics. 1st ed. New York: Springer; 1995. pp. 281-299. DOI: 10.1007/978-1-4612-2544-7_17

[24] Liang J, Parks TW. A translation-invariant wavelet representation algorithm with applications. IEEE Transactions on Signal Processing. 1995;**44**:225-232

[25] Rioul O, Vetterli M. Wavelets and signal processing. IEEE Signal Processing Magazine. 1991;**8**:14-38. DOI: 10.1109/79.91217

[26] Grossmann A, Kronland-Martinet R, Morlet J. Reading and understanding continuous wavelet transforms. In: Combes JM, Grossmann A, Tchamitchian P, editors. Wavelets. Inverse Problems and Theoretical Imaging. Berlin, Springer; 1990. pp. 2-20. DOI: 10.1007/978-3-642-75988-8_1

[27] Liò P, Vannucci M. Finding pathogenicity islands and gene transfer events in genoma data. Bioinformatics. 2000;**16**:932-940. DOI: 10.1093/bioinformatics/16.10.932

[28] Linden R. Técnicas de agrupamento. Revista de Sistemas de Informação da FSMA. 2009;**4**:18-36

[29] Hartigan JA. Clustering Algorithms. 99th ed. New York: John Wiley & Sons; 1975. 369 p

[30] Friedman J, Hastie T, Tibshirani R. Regularization paths for generalized linear models via coordinate descent. Journal of Statistical Software. 2010;**33**:1-22

[31] Hoerl AE, Kennard RW. Ridge regression: Biased estimation for nonorthogonal problems. Technometrics. 1970;**12**:55-67

[32] Piepho HP. Ridge regression and extensions for genome wide selection in maize. Crop Science. 2009;**49**:1165-1176. DOI: 10.2135/cropsci2008.10.0595

[33] Zou H, Hastie T. Regularization and variable selection via the elastic net. Journal of the Royal Statistical Society, Series B: Statistical Methodology. 2005;**67**:301-320. DOI: 10.1111/j.1467-9868.2005.00503.x

[34] Ferreira LM, Sáfadi T, Ferreira JL. Wavelet-domain elastic net for clustering on genomes strains. Genetics and Molecular Biology. 2018;**4**:884-892. DOI: 10.1590/1678-4685-GMB-2018-0035

[35] Ogutu JO, Schulz-Streeck T, Piepho HP. Genomic selection using regularized

linear regression models: Ridge regression, lasso, elastic net and their extensions. BMC Proceedings. 2012;**6**:1-6. DOI: 10.1186/1753-6561-6-S2-S10

[36] Waldmann P, Mészáros G, Gredler B, Fuerst C, Sölkner J. Evaluation of the lasso and the elastic net in genome-wide association studies. Frontiers in Genetics. 2013;**4**:270. DOI: 10.3389/fgene.2013.00270

[37] Mandelbrot BB, Wallis JR. Noah, Joseph, and operational hydrology. Water Resources Research. 1968;**4**:909-918

[38] Mandelbrot BB, Wallis JR. Robustness of the rescaled range R/S in the measurement of noncyclic long run statistical dependence. Water Resources Research. 1969;**5**:967-988

[39] Hurst HE. Long-term storage capacity of reservoirs. Transactions of the American Society of Civil Engineers. 1951;**116**:770-799

[40] Geweke J, Porter-Hudak S. The estimation and application of long memory time series models. Journal of Time Series Analysis. 1983;**4**:221-238. DOI: https://doi.org/10.1111/j.1467-9892.1983.tb00371.x

[41] Beran J, Terrin N. Estimation of the long-memory parameter, based on a multivariate central limit theorem. Journal of Time Series Analysis. 1994;**15**:269-278. DOI: 10.1111/j.1467-9892.1994.tb00192.x

[42] Robinson PM. Gaussian semiparametric estimation of long-range dependence. The Annals of Statistics. 1995;**23**:1630-1661

[43] Riedi RH. Multifractal processes. In: Doukhan P, Oppenheim G, Taqqu MS, editors. Theory and Applications of Long-Range Dependence. 1st ed. Boston: Birkhäuser Boston; 2003. pp. 625-716

[44] Simonsen I, Hansen A, Nes OM. Determination of the Hurst exponent by use of wavelet transforms. Physical Review E. 1998;**58**:2779-2787. DOI: 10.1103/PhysRevE.58.2779

Chapter 2

Bioinformatics Workflows for Genomic Variant Discovery, Interpretation and Prioritization

Osman Ugur Sezerman, Ege Ulgen, Nogayhan Seymen and Ilknur Melis Durasi

Abstract

Next-generation sequencing (NGS) techniques allow high-throughput detection of a vast amount of variations in a cost-efficient manner. However, there still are inconsistencies and debates about how to process and analyse this 'big data'. To accurately extract clinically relevant information from genomics data, choosing appropriate tools, knowing how to best utilize them and interpreting the results correctly is crucial. This chapter reviews state-of-the-art bioinformatics approaches in clinically relevant genomic variant detection. Best practices of reads-to-variant discovery workflows for germline and somatic short genomic variants are presented along with the most commonly utilized tools for each step. Additionally, methods for detecting structural variations are overviewed. Finally, approaches and current guidelines for clinical interpretation of genomic variants are discussed. As emphasized in this chapter, data processing and variant discovery steps are relatively well-understood. The differences in prioritization algorithms on the other hand can be perplexing, thus creating a bottleneck during interpretation. This review aims to shed light on the pros and cons of these differences to help experts give more informed decisions.

Keywords: genomics, NGS, variant discovery

1. Introduction

Whole genome sequencing (WGS) and whole exome sequencing are next-generation sequencing (NGS) technologies that determine the full and protein-coding genomic sequence of an organism, respectively. Deep sequencing of genomes improves understanding of clinical interpretation of genomic variations. Analyzing NGS data with the aim of understanding the impact and the importance of genomic variations in health and disease conditions is crucial for carrying the personalized medicine applications one step further.

One of the main obstacles for reaching the full potential of WES/WGS in personalized medicine is bioinformatics analysis, which mostly requires strong computational power. Analysis of WES/WGS data with publicly or commercially available algorithms and tools require a proper computational infrastructure in addition to an at least basic understanding of NGS technologies. Second, almost all publicly available algorithms and tools focus on a single aspect of the entire process and do not provide a workflow that can aid the researcher from start to finish. Lastly, there are no gold standards for translating WES/WGS into clinical knowledge, since different diseases need different strategies for the basic analysis to obtain the genomic variants as well as further analyses, including disease-specific interpretation and prioritization of the variants.

A comprehensive workflow that can be applied for WES/WGS data analysis is composed of the following steps:

a. Quality control

- Evaluation of the quality of FASTQ data

- Trimming of the low-quality reads and removal of adaptors (if necessary)

b. Sequence alignment

c. Post-alignment processing

- Marking PCR duplicates

- Base quality score recalibration (BQSR)

d. Variant discovery

e. Downstream analyses

- Filtration of genomic variations

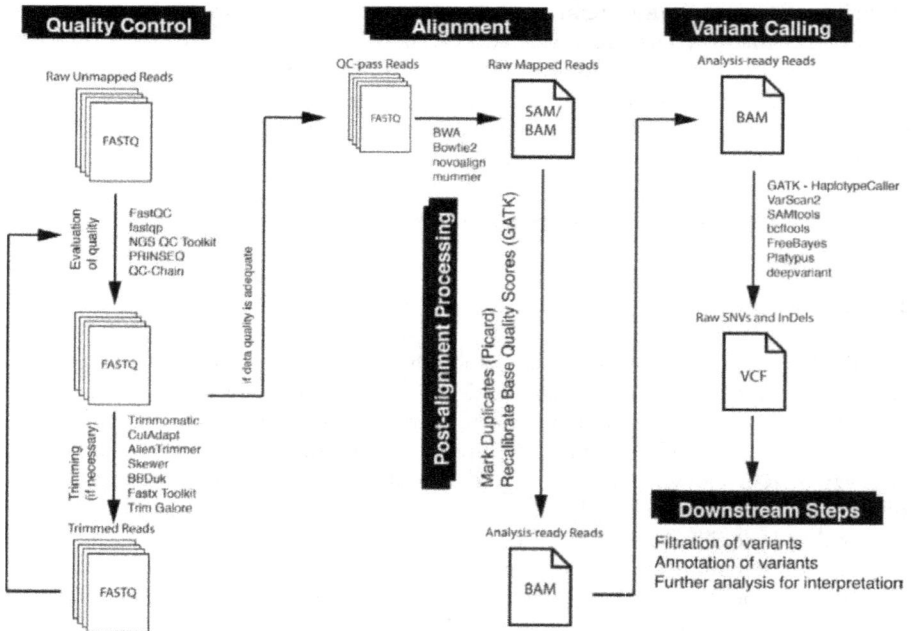

Figure 1.
An example single-sample variant discovery workflow. Each step is labelled in the black rectangles. The most widely used tools for each operation are also presented.

- Annotation via a variant annotation tool

- Interpretation/prioritization of genomic variations

An example reads-to-variants workflow is visualized in **Figure 1**, highlighting the input and output, a brief description, and the tools that can be utilized in each step. While we present the most widely used tools, we would like to emphasize that there are a great variety of tools/algorithms that can be utilized for each process.

Through the rest of this chapter, we give a brief outline of the purpose of each step and try to provide a basic understanding of a state-of-the-art workflow for the detection and interpretation of genomic variations. While there are countless experimental designs, including WES/WGS and targeted (gene panel) sequencing, the workflow presented here is applicable for all designs, occasionally requiring slight modifications. We particularly focus on the detection and interpretation of germline short variants, namely, single nucleotide variations (SNVs) and germline short insertion or deletion events (indels). However, outlines of analyses for somatic variants and for structural variations (SVs) are also presented. Finally, current approaches and tools for clinical interpretation of genomic variations are discussed.

2. Detection of genomic variations

Detection of genomic variations beginning from raw read data is a multistep task that can be executed using numerous tools and resources. The workflow outlined in the introduction section is laid out in detail in this section, including the best practice recommendations and common pitfalls.

2.1 Acquisition of raw read data: the FASTQ file format

The raw data from a sequencing machine are most widely provided as FASTQ files, which include sequence information, similar to FASTA files, but additionally contain further information, including sequence quality information.

A FASTQ file consists of blocks, corresponding to reads, and each block consists of four elements in four lines (**Figure 2**).

The first line contains a sequence identifier and includes an optional description of sequencing information (such as machine ID, lane, tile, etc.). The raw sequence letters are presented in line 2. The third line begins with a "+" sign and optionally contains the same sequence identifier. The last line encodes the quality score for the sequence in line 2 in the form of ASCII characters. While specific scoring measures might differ among platforms, Phred Score (Q_{phred} = -10log$_{10}$P, where P being the probability of misreading any given base) is the most widely used.

2.2 Quality control

In general, the raw sequence data acquired from a sequencing provider is not immediately ready to be used for variant discovery. The first and most important

```
@EAS100R:136:FC706VJ:2:2104:15343:197393 1:Y:18:ATCAG
GATTTGGGGTTCAAAGCAGTATCGATCAAATAGTAAATCCATTTGTTCAACTCACAGTTT
+
!''*(((( ***+ ))%%%++ )(%%%).1***-+*''))**55CCF>>>>>>CCCCCCC65
```

Figure 2.
Example FASTQ file format.

step of the WES/WGS analysis workflow following data acquisition is the quality control (QC) step. QC is the process of improving raw data by removing any identifiable errors from it. By performing QC at the beginning of the analysis, chances encountering any contamination, bias, error, and missing data are minimized.

The QC process is a cyclical process, in which (i) the quality is evaluated, (ii) QC is stopped if the quality is adequate, and (iii) a data altering step (e.g., trimming of low-quality reads, removal of adapters, etc.) is performed, and then the QC is repeated beginning from step (i).

The most commonly used tool for evaluating and visualizing the quality of FASTQ data is FastQC (Babraham Bioinformatics, n.d.), which provides comprehensive information about data quality, including but not limited to per base sequence quality scores, GC content information, sequence duplication levels, and overrepresented sequences (**Figure** 3). Alternatives to FastQC include, but are not limited to, fastqp, NGS QC Toolkit, PRINSEQ, and QC-Chain.

Below, QC approaches for the most commonly encountered data quality issues are discussed: adapter contamination and low-quality measurements toward the 5' and 3' ends of reads.

Adapters are ligated to the 5' and 3' ends of each single DNA molecule during sequencing. These adapter sequences hold barcoding sequences, forward/reverse primers, and the binding sequences to immobilize the fragments to the flow cell and allow bridge amplification. Since the adapter sequences are synthetic and are not seen in any genomic sequence, adapter contamination often leads to NGS alignment errors and an increased number of unaligned reads. Hence, any adapter sequences need to be removed before mapping. In addition to adapter removal, trimming can be performed to discard any low-quality reads, which generally occur at the 5' and 3' ends.

There is an abundance of tools for QC, namely, Trimmomatic [1], CutAdapt [2], AlienTrimmer [3], Skewer [4], BBDuk [5], Fastx Toolkit [6], and Trim Galore [7].

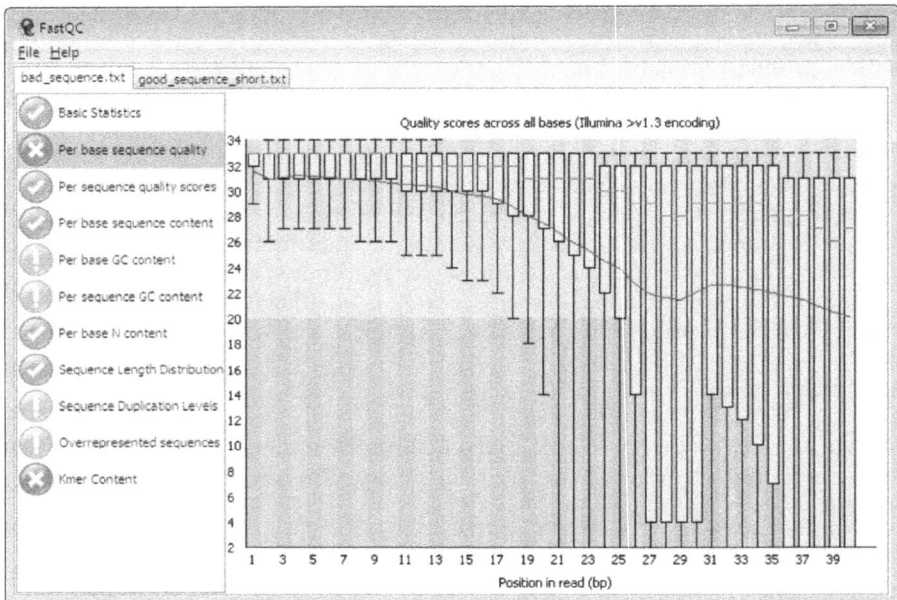

Figure 3.
An example FastQC result.

In addition to these stand-alone tools, R packages for QC, such as PIQA and ShortRead, are also available.

While QC is the most important step of NGS analysis, one must keep in mind that once basic corrections (such as the ones described above) are made, no amount of further QC can produce a radically better outcome. QC cannot simply turn bad data into good data. Moreover, it is also important to remember that because QC may also introduce error that can affect the analysis, it is vital never to perform error correction on data that does not need it.

2.3 Sequence alignment

In order to find the exact locations of reads, each must be aligned to a reference genome. Efficiency and accuracy are crucial in this step because large quantities of reads could take days to align and a low-accuracy alignment would cause inadequate analyses. For humans, the most current and widely used reference sequences are GRCh37 (hg19) and GRCh38 (hg38). Similar to any bioinformatics problem, there are a great number of tools for alignment of sequences to the reference genome, to name a few, BWA [8], Bowtie2 [9], novoalign [10], and mummer [11].

After aligning, a Sequence Alignment Map (SAM) file is produced. This file contains the reads aligned to the reference. The binary version of a SAM file is termed a Binary Alignment Map (BAM) file, and BAM files are utilized for random-access purposes. The SAM/BAM file consists of a header and an alignment section. The header section contains contigs of aligned reference sequence, read groups (carrying platform, library, and sample information), and (optionally) data processing tools applied to the reads. The alignment section includes information on the alignments of reads.

2.4 Post-alignment processing

One of the key steps in any reads-to-variants workflow is post-alignment data processing to produce analysis-ready BAM files. This step includes data clean-up operations to correct for technical biases: marking duplicates and recalibration of base quality scores.

During the preparation of samples for sequencing, PCR duplicates arise at the step of PCR amplification of fragments. Since they share the same sequence and the same alignment position, they can lead to problems in variant detection. For example, during SNV calling, false-positive variants may arise as some alleles may be overrepresented due to amplification biases. To overcome this issue, PCR duplicates are marked with a certain tag using an algorithm (MarkDuplicates) available in the tool Picard [12]. Marking duplicates constitutes a major bottleneck since it involves making a large number of comparisons between all the read pairs. Thus, the majority of the effort in optimizing the runtime of reads-to-variants workflows is focused on this step.

As aforementioned, NGS platforms provide information on the quality of each base that they measure in the Phred Score format. The relationship of a Phred Score with accuracy is straightforward: a Phred Score of 10 represents 90% accuracy, 20 equals 99%, 30 equals 99.9%, and so on. The raw scores produced by the sequencing machine are prone to technical errors, leading to over- or underestimated base quality scores. Base quality score recalibration (BQSR) is a machine learning approach that models these errors empirically and readjusts the base quality scores accordingly. Through this recalibration, more accurate and reliable base quality scores are achieved, which in turn improves the reliability of the downstream steps in further analyses. The most widely used tool for BQSR is provided by the Genome Analysis Toolkit (GATK) [13].

After these post-alignment data processing operations, an analysis-ready BAM file is obtained.

2.5 Short variant discovery

In this section, approaches for the discovery of germline SNV and indels are discussed. In the following sections, approaches for the discovery of somatic short variants and of structural variations are outlined.

Following data processing steps, the reads are ready for downstream analyses, and the following step is most frequently variant calling. Variant calling is the process of identifying differences between the sequencing reads, resulting from NGS experiments and a reference genome. Countless variant callers have been and are being developed for accomplishing this challenging task as alignment and sequencing artifacts complicate the process of variant calling. For recent studies comparing different variant callers, see [14–16]. Methods for detecting short variants can be broadly categorized into "probabilistic methods" and "heuristic-based algorithms." In probabilistic methods, the distribution of the observed data is modeled, and then Bayesian statistics is utilized to calculate genotype probabilities. In contrast, in heuristic-based algorithms, variant calls are made based on a number of heuristic factors, such as read quality cutoffs, minimum allele counts, and bounds on read depth. Whereas heuristic-based algorithms are not as widely used, they can be robust to outlying data that violate the assumptions of probabilistic models.

The most widely used state-of-the-art variant callers include, but are not limited to, GATK-HaplotypeCaller [13], SOAPsnp [17], SAMTools [18], bcftools [18], Strelka [19], FreeBayes [20], Platypus [21], and DeepVariant [22]. We would like to emphasize that for WES/WGS, a combination of different variant callers outperforms any single method [23].

2.6 Filtration of variants

Following the variant calling step, raw SNV and indels in the Variant Call Format (VCF) are obtained. These should then be filtered either through applying hard filters to the data or through a more complex approach such as GATK's Variant Quality Score Recalibration (VQSR).

Hard filtering is applied by filtering via thresholds for metrics such as QualByDepth, FisherStrand, RMSMappingQuality, MappingQualityRankSumTest, ReadPosRankSumTest, and StrandOddsRatio.

VQSR, on the other hand, relies on machine learning to identify annotation profiles of variants that are likely to be real. It requires a large training dataset (minimum 30 WES data, at least one WGS data if possible) and well-curated sets of known variants. The aim is to assign a well-calibrated probability to each variant call to create accurate variant quality scores that are then used for filtering.

The accuracy of variant calling is also affected by coverage. Coverage can be broadly defined as the number of unique reads that include a given nucleotide. Coverage is affected by the accuracy of alignment algorithms and by the "mappability" of reads. Coverage can be utilized for both the filtration of variants and for a general evaluation of the sequencing experiment. Tools for assessing coverage information include GATK [13], BEDTools [24], Sambamba [25], and RefCov [26].

For validation of variants and for detecting sequencing artifacts, Integrative Genomics Viewer (IGV) [27] can be used to visualize the processed reads. In addition to this in silico evaluation, Sanger sequencing can be performed.

2.7 Variant annotation

Variant annotation is yet another critical step in the WES/WGS analysis workflow. The aim of all functional annotation tools is to annotate information of the variant effects/consequences, including but not limited to (i) listing which gene (s)/transcript(s) are affected, (ii) determination of the consequence on protein sequence, (iii) correlation of the variant with known genomic annotations (e.g., coding sequence, intronic sequence, noncoding RNA, regulatory regions, etc.), and (iv) matching known variants found in variant databases (e.g., dbSNP [28], 1000 Genomes Project [29], ExAc [30], gnomAD [31], COSMIC [32], ClinVar [33], etc.). The consequence of each variant is expressed through Sequence Ontology (SO) terms. The severity and impact of these consequences are often indicated using qualifiers (e.g., low, moderate, high).

Many annotation tools utilize the predictions of SNV/indel deleteriousness prediction methods, to name a few, SIFT [34], PolyPhen-2 [35], LRT [36], MutationTaster [37], MutationAssessor [38], FATHMM [39], GERP++ [40], PhyloP [41], SiPhy [42], PANTHER-PSEP [43], CONDEL [44], CADD [45], CHASM [46], CanDrA [47], and VEST [48].

Annotation can have a strong influence on the ultimate conclusions during interpretation of genomic variations as incomplete or incorrect annotation information will result in the researcher/clinician to overlook potentially relevant findings.

Once the analysis-ready VCF is produced, the genomic variants can then be annotated using a variety of tools and a variety of transcript sets. Both the choice of annotation software and transcript set (e.g., RefSeq transcript set [49], Ensembl transcript set [50]) have been shown to be important for variant annotation [51]. The most widely used functional annotation tools include but are not limited to AnnoVar [52], SnpEff [53], Variant Effect Predictor (VEP) [54], GEMINI [55], VarAFT [56], VAAST [57], TransVar [58], MAGI [59], SNPnexus [60], and VarMatch [61]. Below some of the popular tools are briefly described:

AnnoVar: AnnoVar is one of the most popular tools for annotation of SNV and indels. AnnoVar takes a simple text-based format that includes chr, start, end, ref, alt, and optional field(s) as an input. To use AnnoVar, one must convert VCF file format to the AnnoVar input file format. The tool returns a single annotation for each variant. If there exists more than one transcript for a specific variant resulting in different consequences, AnnoVar chooses the transcript according to the gene definition set by the user.

SnpEff: SnpEff is an open-source tool that annotates variants and predicts their effects on genes by using an interval forest approach. SnpEff annotates variants based on their genomic locations such as intronic, untranslated region, upstream, downstream, splice site, or intergenic regions and predicts coding effects. snpEff also generates extensive report files and is easily customizable.

VEP: VEP is an open-source, free-to-use toolset for the analysis, annotation, and prioritization of genomic variants in coding and noncoding regions. VEP is one of the few annotation tools that annotates variants in regulatory regions.

GEnome MINIng (GEMINI): GEMINI is a flexible software package for exploring all forms of human genetic variations. Different from most other annotation tools, GEMINI integrates genetic variation with a set of genome annotations.

While the abovementioned are all variant annotation tools, it might be wise to put GEMINI in a different category as it has other built-in tools to make further analysis of the variants easier.

2.8 Somatic genomic variations

The workflow for identifying somatic short variants (somatic SNV/indels) is nearly identical to the germline short variant discovery workflow (**Figure 4**). However, several differences exist. Firstly, for the discovery of somatic genomic variations, sequencing both tumor tissue and a matched normal sample (blood, adjacent normal tissue, etc.) is mostly (but not necessarily) preferred. The QC, alignment, and post-alignment data processing steps are identical and are performed for both the tumor and normal data, separately. The main difference is the variant calling step, where both the tumor and normal processed read data are utilized to identify somatic SNV/indels, i.e., short variants that are present in the tumor but not in the normal. Some tools (such as GATK-MuTect2) can utilize additional information from a panel of normals, a collection of normal samples (typically larger than 40) that are believed to have no somatic variants, processed in the same manner at each step and the purpose of which is to capture recurrent technical artifacts.

Several tools exist for tumor-normal somatic variant calling, to name a few, GATK - MuTect2 [13], VarScan2 [62], Strelka [19], SomaticSniper [63], SAMtools [18], SomaticSeq [64], FreeBayes [65], CaVEMan [66], and FaSD-somatic [67]. For further information on somatic variant calling, we encourage the reader to refer to a recent and comprehensive review on somatic variant calling algorithms [16].

Filtration of the raw SNV and indels also differs for the somatic workflow. Several different approaches exist for the filtration of raw somatic variants. Most

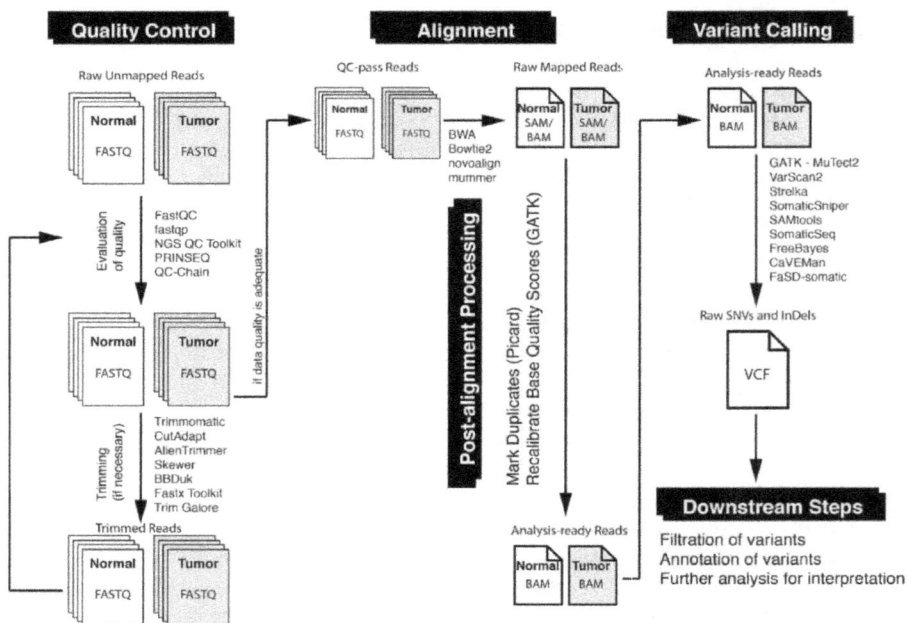

Figure 4.
An example somatic variant discovery workflow. Each step is labelled in the black rectangles. Most widely used tools for each operation are also presented. As can be seen in the diagram, the processing steps until the variant calling step are performed for both the normal and tumor data, separately.

frequently, tumor-specific metrics including the estimation of tumor heterogeneity and cross-sample contamination are used in addition to the aforementioned metrics for detection of sequencing/alignment artifacts.

While all the annotation tools, presented in the "variant annotation" section, can be used to annotate somatic variants, a number of tools that provide cancer-specific annotation in addition to general annotation are available. Two popular examples are Oncotator [68] and CRAVAT [69]. Oncotator, a widely used cancer-specific annotation tool, is often preferred for the annotation of somatic short variants. Oncotator provides variant- and gene-centric information relevant to cancer researchers, utilizing resources including but not limited to the Catalogue of Somatic Mutations in Cancer (COSMIC) [70], the Cancer Gene Census [71], Cancer Cell Line Encyclopedia [72], The Cancer Genome Atlas (TCGA), and Familial Cancer Database [73].

2.9 Structural variations

So far, we focused only on the discovery of small-scale genomic variations (SNVs and indels). There also exist large-scale (1 kb and larger) genomic variations, which either be copy number variations (CNV) or chromosomal rearrangement events (including translocations, inversions, and duplications).

2.9.1 Copy number variations

CNV is a frequent form of critical genetic variation that results in an abnormal number of copies of large genomic regions (either gain or loss events). CNV is clinically relevant, as they may play vital roles in disease processes, especially during oncogenesis. It is possible to detect CNVs using WES/WGS data. Several different approaches exist for this purpose [74]:

i. **Paired-end mapping** strategy detects CNVs through discordantly mapped reads. Tools utilizing this approach include BreakDancer, PEMer, VariationHunter, commonLAW, GASV, and Spanner.

ii. **Split read-based** methods use the incompletely mapped read from each read pair to identify small CNVs. Split read-based tools include AGE, Pindel, SLOPE, and SRiC.

iii. **Read depth-based** approach detects CNV by counting the number of reads mapped to each genomic region. Tools using this approach include GATK, SegSeq, CNV-seq, RDXplorer, BIC-seq, CNAseq, cn.MOPS, jointSLM, ReadDepth, rSW-seq, CNVnator, CNVnorm, CMDS, mrCaNaVar, CNVeM, and cnvHMM.

iv. **Assembly-based** approach detects CNVs by mapping contigs to the reference genome. Tools using this approach include Magnolya, Cortex assembler, and TIGRA-SV.

v. **Combinatorial** approach combines read depth and paired-end mapping information to detect CNVs. Tools using this approach include NovelSeq, HYDRA, CNVer, GASVPro, Genome STRiP, SVDetect, inGAP-sv, and SVseq.

In addition to the noise and artifacts caused by WES/WGS, tumor complexity (the strongest factor being tumor heterogeneity) makes the detection of somatic

CNVs more challenging. To overcome this challenge, numerous tools have been developed. Widely used tools for detecting specifically somatic CNVs include ADTEx [75], CONTRA [76], cn.MOPS [77], ExomeCNV [78], VarScan2 [62], SynthEx [79], Control-FREEC [80], GATK [13], and CloneCNA [81].

2.9.2 Chromosomal rearrangements

Chromosomal rearrangements are variations in chromosome structure whose impact on genetic diversity and disease susceptibility has become increasingly evident [82]. Per SO, numerous types of rearrangements exist: duplication, deletion, insertion, mobile element insertion, novel sequence insertion, tandem duplication, inversion, intrachromosomal breakpoint, interchromosomal breakpoint, translocation, and complex SVs. Similar to CNV detection, there are multiple approaches for rearrangement detection: read-pair, split-read, read-depth, and assembly approaches. The underlying aims of each of these approaches are very similar to those for CNV detection. As for CNV detection, countless tools have been developed for the detection of rearrangement variations, including but not limited to Breakdancer [83], GRIMM [84], LUMPY [85], BreaKmer [86], BreakSeek [87], CREST [88], DELLY [89], HYDRA [90], MultiBreak-SV [91], Pindel [92], SoftSearch [93], SVdetect [94], and TIGRA-SV [95].

Lastly, we would like to point out that long reads (enabled by the emergence of so-called third-generation sequencing technologies) allow for more accurate and reliable determination of SVs with the development of novel algorithms that specifically exploits these long reads [96].

3. Clinical interpretation of genomic variations

Perhaps the most challenging process in WES/WGS analysis is the clinical interpretation of genomic variations. While WES/WGS is rapidly becoming a routine approach for the diagnosis of monogenic and complex disorders and personalized treatment of such disorders, it is still challenging to interpret the vast amount of genomic variation data detected through WES/WGS [97].

There exist numerous standardized widely accepted guidelines for the evaluation of genomic variations obtained through NGS such as the American College of Medical Genetics and Genomics (ACMG), the EuroGentest, and the European Society of Human Genetics guidelines. These provide standards and guidelines for the interpretation of genomic variations and include evidence-based recommendations on aspects including the use of literature and database and the use of in silico predictors, criteria for variant interpretation, and reporting.

In addition to variant-dependent annotation such as allele frequency (e.g., in 1000 Genomes [29], ExAc [30], gnomAD [31]), the predicted effect on protein and evolutionary conservation, disease-dependent inquiries such as mode of inheritance, co-segregation of variant with disease within families, prior association of the variant/gene with disease, investigation of clinical actionability, and pathway-based analysis are required for the interpretation of genomic variants.

Databases such as ClinVar [33], HGV databases [98], OMIM [99], COSMIC [100], and CIViC [101] are excellent resources that can aid interpretations of clinical significance of germline and somatic variants for reported conditions. The availability of shared genetic data in such databases makes it possible to identify patients with similar conditions and aid the clinician to make a conclusive diagnosis.

While one may perform interpretation of genomic variations completely manually after annotation and filtering of variants, there are several tools to aid in interpretation and prioritization of these variants, including Ingenuity Variant Analysis [102], BaseSpace Variant Interpreter [103], VariantStudio [104], KGGSeq [105], PhenoTips [106], VarElect [107], PhenoVar [108], InterVar [109], VarSifter [110], eXtasy [111], VAAST [57], and Exomiser [112]. For personalized oncology purposes, numerous cancer-specific tools exist, specifically developed to determine driver genes/mutations as well as to aid in interpretation of somatic variants. Some of the most widely used somatic interpretation tools are PHIAL, PCGR, and HitWalker2.

Pathway analysis is another powerful component that can enhance the interpretation of genomic variations. Pathway analysis can be broadly defined as a group of methods incorporating biological information from public databases to simplify analysis by grouping long lists of genes into smaller sets of related genes (for a comprehensive review on pathway analysis, see [113]). Pathway analysis improves the detection of causal variants by incorporating biologic insight. The clinician can gain a better understanding of the functions of rare genetic variants of unknown clinical significance in the context of biological pathways. While the gene carrying the variant may not be related to the phenotype, its associated genes in the pathway might be causally related to the phenotype at hand. Moreover, through pathway analysis, the role of multiple variants and their interaction on disease formation can be discovered.

Countless tools for pathway analysis exist. Some of the widely used pathway analysis tools are GSEA [114], DAVID [115], IPA [116], SPIA [117], pathfindR [118], enrichr [119], reactomePA [120], MetaCore [121], and PathVisio [122]. Additionally, many different pathway resources exist, the most popular of which are Kyoto Encyclopedia of Genes and Genomes [123], Reactome [124], WikiPathways [125], MSigDb [126], STRINGDB [127], Pathway Commons [128], Ingenuity Knowledge Base [129], and Pathway Studio [130].

In silico interpretation often fails to provide conclusive evidence for pathogenicity of genomic variations [131]. Furthermore, these in silico interpretations are mostly only well-supported predictions (this is especially true for VUS). It is therefore vital to perform functional validation to understand the functional consequences of genetic variants, provide a conclusive diagnosis, and inform the patient on the disease course. Functional validation can be performed using different model systems (e.g., patient cells, model cell lines, model organisms, induced pluripotent stem cells) and performing the suitable type of assay (e.g., genetic rescue, overexpression, biomarker analysis).

4. Conclusion

The advancements in NGS, the increasing availability and applicability of WES/WGS analysis due to decrease in cost, and the development of countless bioinformatics methods and resources enabled the usage of WES/WGS to detect, interpret, and validate genomic variations in the clinical setting.

As we attempted to describe in this chapter, WES/WGS analysis is challenging, and there are a great number of tools for each step of variation discovery. Therefore, one must carefully evaluate the advantages and disadvantages and suitability of different tools (depending on the specific application) before adapting the "optimal" one into the variation discovery workflow. An optimal and coordinated combination of tools is required to identify the different types of genomic variants, described here. On the one hand, an efficient analysis strategy needs to adopt one or more methods for the detection of each type of variant and, on the other hand, needs to integrate results for the different types of variants into a single comprehensive solution.

We attempted to describe the best practices for variant discovery, outlining the fundamental aspects. We hope to have provided a basic understanding of WES/WGS analysis as we believe awareness of the steps involved as well as the challenges involved at each step is important to understand how each piece may affect the downstream steps (and eventually affect interpretation). As emphasized throughout the chapter, substantial (or even minor) changes at any step can fundamentally alter the outcomes in the later stages.

While there is no definite gold standard for the interpretation of genomic variations, we attempted to briefly describe the currently available and widely used guidelines, tools, and resources for clinical evaluation of genomic variations.

In the following years, with the advancements in bioinformatics, increasing cooperation between the clinician and bioinformatician and large-scale efforts (such as IRDiRC [132], TCGA [133], and ICGC [134]), we expect that a greater focus will be on developing novel tools for clinical interpretation of genomic variations. Cooperation between multiple disciplines is vital to improve the existing approaches as well as to develop novel approaches and resources.

Author details

Osman Ugur Sezerman*, Ege Ulgen, Nogayhan Seymen and Ilknur Melis Durasi
Department of Biostatistics and Medical Informatics, Acibadem Mehmet Ali Aydinlar University, Istanbul, Turkey

*Address all correspondence to: sezermanu@gmail.com

IntechOpen

References

[1] Bolger AM, Lohse M, Usadel B. Trimmomatic: A flexible trimmer for illumina sequence data. Bioinformatics. 2014;**30**(15):2114-2120

[2] Martin M. Cutadapt removes adapter sequences from high-throughput sequencing reads. EMBnet.Journal. 2011;**17**(1):10-12

[3] Criscuolo A, Brisse S. AlienTrimmer: A tool to quickly and accurately trim off multiple short contaminant sequences from high-throughput sequencing reads. Genomics. 2013;**102**(5-6): 500-506

[4] Jiang H, Lei R, Ding SW, Zhu S. Skewer: A fast and accurate adapter trimmer for next-generation sequencing paired-end reads. BMC Bioinformatics. 2014;**15**:182

[5] Available from: https://jgi.doe.gov/data-and-tools/bbtools/

[6] Available from: http://hannonlab.cshl.edu/fastx_toolkit/

[7] Available from: https://github.com/FelixKrueger/TrimGalore

[8] Li H, Durbin R. Fast and accurate short read alignment with Burrows-Wheeler transform. Bioinformatics. 2009;**25**(14):1754-1760

[9] Langmead B, Salzberg SL. Fast gapped-read alignment with Bowtie 2. Nature Methods. 2012;**9**(4):357-359

[10] Available from: http://novocraft.com/

[11] Marçais G, Delcher AL, Phillippy AM, Coston R, Salzberg SL, Zimin A. MUMmer4: A fast and versatile genome alignment system. PLoS Computational Biology. 2018;**14**(1):e1005944

[12] Available from: http://broadinstitute.github.io/picard/

[13] Mckenna A, Hanna M, Banks E, et al. The genome analysis toolkit: A MapReduce framework for analyzing next-generation DNA sequencing data. Genome Research. 2010;**20**(9): 1297-1303

[14] Sandmann S, De graaf AO, Karimi M, et al. Evaluating variant calling tools for non-matched next-generation sequencing data. Scientific Reports. 2017;**7**:43169

[15] Bian X, Zhu B, Wang M, et al. Comparing the performance of selected variant callers using synthetic data and genome segmentation. BMC Bioinformatics. 2018;**19**(1):429

[16] Xu C. A review of somatic single nucleotide variant calling algorithms for next-generation sequencing data. Computational and Structural Biotechnology Journal. 2018;**16**:15-24. DOI: 10.1016/j.csbj.2018.01.003

[17] Li R, Li Y, Fang X, et al. SNP detection for massively parallel whole-genome resequencing. Genome Research. 2009;**19**(6):1124-1132

[18] Li H, Handsaker B, Wysoker A, et al. The sequence alignment/map format and SAMtools. Bioinformatics. 2009;**25**(16):2078-2079

[19] Saunders CT, Wong WS, Swamy S, Becq J, Murray LJ, Cheetham RK. Strelka: Accurate somatic small-variant calling from sequenced tumor-normal sample pairs. Bioinformatics. 2012; **28**(14):1811-1817

[20] Available from: https://arxiv.org/abs/1207.3907

[21] Rimmer A, Phan H, Mathieson I, et al. Integrating mapping-, assembly- and haplotype-based approaches for calling variants in clinical sequencing

applications. Nature Genetics. 2014; **46**(8):912-918

[22] Poplin R, Chang P-C, Alexander D, et al. A universal SNP and small-indel variant caller using deep neural networks. Nature Biotechnology. 2018; **36**(10):983-987. DOI: 10.1038/nbt.4235

[23] Bao R, Huang L, Andrade J, et al. Review of current methods, applications, and data management for the bioinformatics analysis of whole exome sequencing. Cancer Informatics. 2014;**13**(Suppl 2):67-82

[24] Quinlan AR, Hall IM. BEDTools: A flexible suite of utilities for comparing genomic features. Bioinformatics. 2010; **26**(6):841-842

[25] Tarasov A, Vilella AJ, Cuppen E, Nijman IJ, Prins P. Sambamba: Fast processing of NGS alignment formats. Bioinformatics. 2015;**31**(12):2032-2034

[26] Available from: http://gmt.genome. wustl.edu/gmt-refcov

[27] Robinson JT, Thorvaldsdóttir H, Winckler W, et al. Integrative genomics viewer. Nature Biotechnology. 2011; **29**(1):24-26

[28] Sherry ST, Ward MH, Kholodov M, et al. dbSNP: The NCBI database of genetic variation. Nucleic Acids Research. 2001;**29**(1):308-311

[29] Auton A, Brooks LD, Durbin RM, et al. A global reference for human genetic variation. Nature. 2015; **526**(7571):68-74

[30] Lek M, Karczewski KJ, Minikel EV, et al. Analysis of protein-coding genetic variation in 60,706 humans. Nature. 2016;**536**(7616):285-291

[31] Available from: https://gnomad.b roadinstitute.org/

[32] Tate JG, Bamford S, Jubb HC, et al. COSMIC: The catalogue of somatic mutations in cancer. Nucleic Acids Research. 2019;**47**(D1):D941-D947

[33] Landrum MJ, Lee JM, Riley GR, et al. ClinVar: Public archive of relationships among sequence variation and human phenotype. Nucleic Acids Research. 2014;**42**(Database issue): D980-D985

[34] Ng PC, Henikoff S. SIFT: Predicting amino acid changes that affect protein function. Nucleic Acids Research. 2003; **31**(13):3812-3814

[35] Adzhubei IA, Schmidt S, Peshkin L, et al. A method and server for predicting damaging missense mutations. Nature Methods. 2010;**7**(4):248-249

[36] Chun S, Fay JC. Identification of deleterious mutations within three human genomes. Genome Research. 2009;**19**(9):1553-1561

[37] Schwarz JM, Rödelsperger C, Schuelke M, Seelow D. MutationTaster evaluates disease-causing potential of sequence alterations. Nature Methods. 2010;**7**:575-576

[38] Reva B, Antipin Y, Sander C. Predicting the functional impact of protein mutations: Application to cancer genomics. Nucleic Acids Research. 2011; **39**(17):e118

[39] Shihab HA, Gough J, Cooper DN, et al. Predicting the functional, molecular, and phenotypic consequences of amino acid substitutions using hidden Markov models. Human Mutation. 2013;**34**(1): 57-65

[40] Davydov EV, Goode DL, Sirota M, Cooper GM, Sidow A, Batzoglou S. Identifying a high fraction of the human genome to be under selective constraint using GERP++. PLoS Computational Biology. 2010;**6**(12):e1001025

[41] Pollard KS, Hubisz MJ, Rosenbloom KR, Siepel A. Detection of nonneutral

substitution rates on mammalian phylogenies. Genome Research. 2010; **20**(1):110-121

[42] Garber M, Guttman M, Clamp M, Zody MC, Friedman N, Xie X. Identifying novel constrained elements by exploiting biased substitution patterns. Bioinformatics. 2009;**25**(12): i54-i62

[43] Tang H, Thomas PD. PANTHER-PSEP: Predicting disease-causing genetic variants using position-specific evolutionary preservation. Bioinformatics. 2016;**32**(14):2230-2232

[44] González-pérez A, López-bigas N. Improving the assessment of the outcome of nonsynonymous SNVs with a consensus deleteriousness score, Condel. American Journal of Human Genetics. 2011;**88**(4):440-449

[45] Rentzsch P, Witten D, Cooper GM, Shendure J, Kircher M. CADD: Predicting the deleteriousness of variants throughout the human genome. Nucleic Acids Research. 2019;**47**(D1): D886-D894

[46] Wong WC, Kim D, Carter H, Diekhans M, Ryan MC, Karchin R. CHASM and SNVBox: Toolkit for detecting biologically important single nucleotide mutations in cancer. Bioinformatics. 2011;**27**(15):2147-2148

[47] Mao Y, Chen H, Liang H, Meric-bernstam F, Mills GB, Chen K. CanDrA: Cancer-specific driver missense mutation annotation with optimized features. PLoS One. 2013;**8**(10):e77945

[48] Carter H, Douville C, Yeo G, Stenson PD, Cooper DN, Karchin R. Identifying Mendelian disease genes with the variant effect scoring tool. BMC Genomics. 2013;**14**(3):1-16

[49] O'leary NA, Wright MW, Brister JR, et al. Reference sequence (RefSeq) database at NCBI: Current status,

taxonomic expansion, and functional annotation. Nucleic Acids Research. 2016;**44**(D1):D733-D745

[50] Zerbino DR, Achuthan P, Akanni W, et al. Ensembl 2018. Nucleic Acids Research. 2018;**46**(D1):D754-D761

[51] Mccarthy DJ, Humburg P, Kanapin A, et al. Choice of transcripts and software has a large effect on variant annotation. Genome Medicine. 2014; **6**(3):26

[52] Wang K, Li M, Hakonarson H. ANNOVAR: Functional annotation of genetic variants from next-generation sequencing data. Nucleic Acids Research. 2010;**38**:e164

[53] Cingolani P, Platts A, Wang le L, et al. A program for annotating and predicting the effects of single nucleotide polymorphisms, SnpEff: SNPs in the genome of Drosophila melanogaster strain w1118; iso-2; iso-3. Fly (Austin). 2012;**6**(2):80-92

[54] Mclaren W, Gil L, Hunt SE, et al. The Ensembl variant effect predictor. Genome Biology. 2016;**17**(1):122

[55] Paila U, Chapman BA, Kirchner R, Quinlan AR. GEMINI: Integrative exploration of genetic variation and genome annotations. PLoS Computational Biology. 2013;**9**(7): e1003153

[56] Desvignes JP, Bartoli M, Delague V, et al. VarAFT: A variant annotation and filtration system for human next generation sequencing data. Nucleic Acids Research. 2018;**46**(W1):W545-W553

[57] Hu H, Huff CD, Moore B, Flygare S, Reese MG, Yandell M. VAAST 2.0: Improved variant classification and disease-gene identification using a conservation-controlled amino acid substitution matrix. Genetic Epidemiology. 2013;**37**(6):622-634

[58] Zhou W, Chen T, Chong Z, et al. TransVar: A multilevel variant annotator for precision genomics. Nature Methods. 2015;**12**(11):1002-1003

[59] Leiserson MD, Gramazio CC, Hu J, Wu HT, Laidlaw DH, Raphael BJ. MAGI: Visualization and collaborative annotation of genomic aberrations. Nature Methods. 2015;**12**(6):483-484

[60] Dayem Ullah AZ, Oscanoa J, Wang J, Nagano A, Lemoine NR, Chelala C. SNPnexus: Assessing the functional relevance of genetic variation to facilitate the promise of precision medicine. Nucleic Acids Research. 2018; **46**(W1):W109-W113

[61] Sun C, Medvedev P. VarMatch: Robust matching of small variant datasets using flexible scoring schemes. Bioinformatics. 2017;**33**(9):1301-1308

[62] Koboldt DC, Zhang Q, Larson DE, et al. VarScan 2: Somatic mutation and copy number alteration discovery in cancer by exome sequencing. Genome Research. 2012;**22**(3):568-576

[63] Larson DE, Harris CC, Chen K, et al. SomaticSniper: Identification of somatic point mutations in whole genome sequencing data. Bioinformatics. 2012; **28**(3):311-317

[64] Fang LT, Afshar PT, Chhibber A, Mohiyuddin M, Fan Y, Mu JC, et al. An ensemble approach to accurately detect somatic mutations using SomaticSeq. Genome Biology. 2015;**16**:197

[65] Available from: http://arxiv.org/abs/1207.3907

[66] Stephens PJ et al. The landscape of cancer genes and mutational processes in breast cancer. Nature. 2012;**486**: 400-404

[67] Wang W, Wang P, Xu F, Luo R, Wong MP, Lam T-W. FaSD-somatic: A fast and accurate somatic SNV detection algorithm for cancer genome sequencing data. Bioinformatics. 2014; **30**(17):2498-2500

[68] Ramos AH, Lichtenstein L, Gupta M, Lawrence MS, Pugh TJ, Saksena G, et al. Oncotator: Cancer variant annotation tool. Human Mutation. 2015; **36**(4):E2423-E24E9. pmid: 25703262

[69] Douville C, Carter H, Kim R, et al. CRAVAT: Cancer-related analysis of variants toolkit. Bioinformatics. 2013; **29**(5):647-648

[70] Forbes SA, Beare D, Boutselakis H, et al. COSMIC: Somatic cancer genetics at high-resolution. Nucleic Acids Research. 2016;**45**(D1):D777-D783

[71] Futreal PA, Andrew Futreal P, Coin L, Marshall M, Down T, Hubbard T, et al. A census of human cancer genes. Nature Reviews. Cancer. 2004;**4**:177-183

[72] Barretina J, Caponigro G, Stransky N, et al. The cancer cell line encyclopedia enables predictive modelling of anticancer drug sensitivity. Nature. 2012;**483**(7391):603-607. Published 2012 Mar 28. DOI: 10.1038/nature11003

[73] Sijmons RH. Identifying Patients with Familial Cancer Syndromes. 2010 Feb 27 [Updated 2010 Feb 27]. In: Riegert-Johnson DL, Boardman LA, Hefferon T, et al., editors. Cancer Syndromes [Internet]. Bethesda (MD): National Center for Biotechnology Information (US); 2009. Available from: https://www.ncbi.nlm.nih.gov/books/NBK45295/

[74] Zhao M, Wang Q, Wang Q, Jia P, Zhao Z. Computational tools for copy number variation (CNV) detection using next-generation sequencing data: Features and perspectives. BMC Bioinformatics. 2013;**14**(11):S1

[75] Amarasinghe KC, Li J, Hunter SM, et al. Inferring copy number and

genotype in tumour exome data. BMC Genomics. 2014;**15**:732

[76] Hooghe B, Hulpiau P, van Roy F, De Bleser P. ConTra: A promoter alignment analysis tool for identification of transcription factor binding sites across species. Nucleic Acids Research. 2008; **36**:W128-W132

[77] Klambauer G, Schwarzbauer K, Mayr A, et al. cn.MOPS: Mixture of Poissons for discovering copy number variations in next-generation sequencing data with a low false discovery rate. Nucleic Acids Research. 2012;**40**(9):e69

[78] Sathirapongsasuti JF, Lee H, Horst BA, et al. Exome sequencing-based copy-number variation and loss of heterozygosity detection: ExomeCNV. Bioinformatics. 2011;**27**(19):2648-2654

[79] Silva GO, Siegel MB, Mose LE, et al. SynthEx: A synthetic-normal-based DNA sequencing tool for copy number alteration detection and tumor heterogeneity profiling. Genome Biology. 2017;**18**(1):66

[80] Boeva V, Popova T, Bleakley K, et al. Control-FREEC: A tool for assessing copy number and allelic content using next-generation sequencing data. Bioinformatics. 2012; **28**(3):423-425

[81] Yu Z, Li A, Wang M. CloneCNA: Detecting subclonal somatic copy number alterations in heterogeneous tumor samples from whole-exome sequencing data. BMC Bioinformatics. 2016;**17**:310

[82] Sedlazeck FJ, Dhroso A, Bodian DL, Paschall J, Hermes F, Zook JM. Tools for annotation and comparison of structural variation. F1000Res. 2017;**6**:1795

[83] Fan X, Abbott TE, Larson D, Chen K. BreakDancer: Identification of genomic structural variation from paired-end read mapping. Current Protocols in Bioinformatics. 2014;**45**: 15.6.1-15.611

[84] Tesler G. GRIMM: Genome rearrangements web server. Bioinformatics. 2002;**18**(3):492-493

[85] Layer RM, Chiang C, Quinlan AR, Hall IM. LUMPY: A probabilistic framework for structural variant discovery. Genome Biology. 2014;**15**(6): R84

[86] Abo RP, Ducar M, Garcia EP, et al. BreaKmer: Detection of structural variation in targeted massively parallel sequencing data using kmers. Nucleic Acids Research. 2014;**43**(3):e19

[87] Zhao H, Zhao F. BreakSeek: A breakpoint-based algorithm for full spectral range INDEL detection. Nucleic Acids Research. 2015;**43**(14):6701-6713

[88] Wang J, Mullighan CG, Easton J, et al. CREST maps somatic structural variation in cancer genomes with base-pair resolution. Nature Methods. 2011; **8**(8):652-654. Published 2011 Jun 12. DOI: 10.1038/nmeth.1628

[89] Rausch T, Zichner T, Schlattl A, Stütz AM, Benes V, Korbel JO. DELLY: Structural variant discovery by integrated paired-end and split-read analysis. Bioinformatics. 2012;**28**(18): i333-i339

[90] Miller PL, Blumenfrucht SJ, Rose JR, et al. HYDRA: A knowledge acquisition tool for expert systems that critique medical workup. Medical Decision Making. 1987;**7**(1):12-21

[91] Ritz A, Bashir A, Sindi S, Hsu D, Hajirasouliha I, Raphael BJ. Characterization of structural variants with single molecule and hybrid sequencing approaches. Bioinformatics. 2014;**30**(24):3458-3466

[92] Ye K, Schulz MH, Long Q, Apweiler R, Ning Z. Pindel: A pattern growth

approach to detect break points of large deletions and medium sized insertions from paired-end short reads. Bioinformatics. 2009;**25**(21):2865-2871

[93] Hart SN, Sarangi V, Moore R, et al. SoftSearch: Integration of multiple sequence features to identify breakpoints of structural variations. PLoS One. 2013;**8**(12):e83356

[94] Zeitouni B, Boeva V, Janoueix-Lerosey I, et al. SVDetect: A tool to identify genomic structural variations from paired-end and mate-pair sequencing data. Bioinformatics. 2010; **26**(15):1895-1896

[95] Chen K, Chen L, Fan X, Wallis J, Ding L, Weinstock G. TIGRA: A targeted iterative graph routing assembler for breakpoint assembly. Genome Research. 2014;**24**(2):310-317

[96] Guan P, Sung WK. Structural variation detection using next-generation sequencing data: A comparative technical review. Methods. 2016;**102**:36-49

[97] Sayitoğlu M. Clinical interpretation of genomic variations. Turkish Journal of Haematology. 2016;**33**(3):172-179

[98] Freeman PJ, Hart RK, Gretton LJ, Brookes AJ, Dalgleish R. VariantValidator: Accurate validation, mapping, and formatting of sequence variation descriptions. Human Mutation. 2017;**39**(1):61-68

[99] Hamosh A, Scott AF, Amberger J, Bocchini C, Valle D, McKusick VA. Online Mendelian Inheritance in Man (OMIM), a knowledgebase of human genes and genetic disorders. Nucleic Acids Research. 2002;**30**(1):52-55

[100] Bamford S, Dawson E, Forbes S, et al. The COSMIC (Catalogue of Somatic Mutations in Cancer) database and website. British Journal of Cancer. 2004;**91**(2):355-358

[101] Griffith M, Spies NC, Krysiak K, et al. CIViC is a community knowledgebase for expert crowdsourcing the clinical interpretation of variants in cancer. Nature Genetics. 2017;**49**(2):170-174

[102] Available from: www.ingenuity.com

[103] Available from: https://www.illumina.com/products/by-type/informatics-products/basespace-variant-interpreter.html

[104] Available from: https://www.bioz.com/result/VariantStudio%20variant/product/Illumina

[105] Li MX, Gui HS, Kwan JS, Bao SY, Sham PC. A comprehensive framework for prioritizing variants in exome sequencing studies of Mendelian diseases. Nucleic Acids Research. 2012; **40**(7):e53

[106] Girdea M, Dumitriu S, Fiume M, et al. PhenoTips: Patient phenotyping software for clinical and research use. Human Mutation. 2013;**34**(8):1057-1065

[107] Stelzer G, Plaschkes I, Oz-levi D, et al. VarElect: The phenotype-based variation prioritizer of the GeneCards Suite. BMC Genomics. 2016;**17**(Suppl 2):444

[108] Trakadis YJ, Buote C, Therriault JF, Jacques PÉ, Larochelle H, Lévesque S. PhenoVar: A phenotype-driven approach in clinical genomics for the diagnosis of polymalformative syndromes. BMC Medical Genomics. 2014;**7**:22. Published 2014 May 12. DOI: 10.1186/1755-8794-7-22

[109] Li Q, Wang K. InterVar: Clinical interpretation of genetic variants by the 2015 ACMG-AMP guidelines. American Journal of Human Genetics. 2017; **100**(2):267-280

[110] Teer JK, Green ED, Mullikin JC, Biesecker LG. VarSifter: Visualizing and

analyzing exome-scale sequence variation data on a desktop computer. Bioinformatics. 2011;**28**(4):599-600

[111] Sifrim A, Popovic D, Tranchevent LC, Ardeshirdavani A, Sakai R, Konings P, et al. eXtasy: Variant prioritization by genomic data fusion. Nature Methods. 2013;**10**(11):1083-1084. DOI: 10.1038/nmeth.2656

[112] Smedley D, Jacobsen JO, Jäger M, et al. Next-generation diagnostics and disease-gene discovery with the Exomiser. Nature Protocols. 2015;**10**(12):2004-2015

[113] García-Campos MA, Espinal-Enríquez J, Hernández-Lemus E. Pathway analysis: State of the art. Frontiers in Physiology. 2015;**6**:383. doi: 10.3389/fphys.2015.00383

[114] Powers RK, Goodspeed A, Pielke-Lombardo H, Tan AC, Costello JC. GSEA-InContext: Identifying novel and common patterns in expression experiments. Bioinformatics. 2018; **34**(13):i555-i564

[115] Dennis G, Sherman BT, Hosack DA, et al. DAVID: Database for annotation, visualization, and integrated discovery. Genome Biology. 2003;**4**(9): R60

[116] Yu J, Gu X, Yi S. Ingenuity pathway analysis of gene expression profiles in distal Nerve stump following nerve injury: Insights into Wallerian degeneration. Frontiers in Cellular Neuroscience. 2016;**10**:274. Published 2016 Dec 6. DOI: 10.3389/fncel.2016.00274

[117] Tarca AL, Draghici S, Khatri P, et al. A novel signaling pathway impact analysis. Bioinformatics. 2008;**25**(1): 75-82

[118] Ulgen E, Ozisik O, Sezerman OU. pathfindR: An R Package for Pathway Enrichment Analysis Utilizing Active Subnetworks. bioRxiv. 2018

[119] Kuleshov MV, Jones MR, Rouillard AD, et al. Enrichr: A comprehensive gene set enrichment analysis web server 2016 update. Nucleic Acids Research. 2016;**44**(W1):W90-W97

[120] Yu G, HeReactomePA Q-Y. An R/Bioconductor package for reactome pathway analysis and visualization. Molecular BioSystems. 2016;**12**:477-479

[121] Available from: https://clarivate.com/products/metacore/

[122] Kutmon M, Van iersel MP, Bohler A, et al. PathVisio 3: An extendable pathway analysis toolbox. PLoS Computational Biology. 2015;**11**(2): e1004085

[123] Kanehisa M, Goto S. KEGG: Kyoto encyclopedia of genes and genomes. Nucleic Acids Research. 2000;**28**(1): 27-30

[124] Croft D, O'Kelly G, Wu G, et al. Reactome: A database of reactions, pathways and biological processes. Nucleic Acids Research. 2010;**39** (Database issue):D691-D697

[125] Kelder T, van Iersel MP, Hanspers K, et al. WikiPathways: Building research communities on biological pathways. Nucleic Acids Research. 2011; **40**(Database issue):D1301-D1307

[126] Liberzon A, Subramanian A, Pinchback R, Thorvaldsdóttir H, Tamayo P, Mesirov JP. Molecular signatures database (MSigDB) 3.0. Bioinformatics. 2011;**27**(12):1739-1740

[127] Szklarczyk D, Morris JH, Cook H, et al. The STRING database in 2017: Quality-controlled protein-protein association networks, made broadly accessible. Nucleic Acids Research. 2016;**45**(D1):D362-D368

[128] Cerami EG, Gross BE, Demir E, et al. Pathway commons, a web resource

for biological pathway data. Nucleic
Acids Research. 2010;**39**(Database
issue):D685-D690

[129] Available from: http://www.inge
nuity.com/

[130] Nikitin A, Egorov S, Daraselia N,
Mazo I. Pathway studio—The analysis
and navigation of molecular networks.
Bioinformatics. 2003;**19**(16):2155-2157

[131] Rodenburg RJ. The functional
genomics laboratory: Functional
validation of genetic variants. Journal of
Inherited Metabolic Disease. 2018;
41(3):297-307

[132] Austin CP, Cutillo CM, Lau LPL,
et al. Future of rare diseases research
2017–2027: An IRDiRC perspective.
Clinical and Translational Science. 2018;
11(1):21-27

[133] Available from: https://cancerge
nome.nih.gov/

[134] Zhang J, Baran J, Cros A, et al.
International cancer genome
consortium data portal—A one-stop
shop for cancer genomics data.
Database: The Journal of Biological
Databases and Curation. 2011;**2011**:
bar026

Orienting Future Trends in Local Ancestry Deconvolution Models to Optimally Decipher Admixed Individual Genome Variations

Gaston K. Mazandu, Ephifania Geza, Milaine Seuneu and Emile R. Chimusa

Abstract

Rapid advances in sequencing and genotyping technologies have significantly contributed to shaping the area of medical and population genetics. Several thousand genomes are completed with millions of variants identified in the human deoxyribonucleic acid (DNA) sequences. These genomic variations highly influence changes in phenotypic manifestations and physiological functions of different individuals or population groups. Of particular importance are variations introduced by admixture event, contributing significantly to a remarkable phenotypic variability with medical and/or evolutionary implications. In this case, knowledge of local ancestry estimates and date of admixture is of utmost importance for a better understanding of genomic variation patterns throughout modern human evolution and adaptive processes. In this chapter, we survey existing local ancestry deconvolution and dating admixture event models to identify possible gaps that still need to be filled and orient future trends in designing more effective models, which account for current challenges and produce more accurate and biological relevant estimates.

Keywords: genomic variations, admixture, local ancestry, dating admixture event, linkage disequilibrium

1. Introduction

Today, advances in high-throughput technologies have generated huge amounts of human genomics data in public domains. These data are useful for medical and population genetics to understand the population history, human evolution and demographics, susceptibility to disease, and response to drug. Over time, humanity has experienced the exchange of genetic materials across populations, mainly due to population migrations [1], which have led to wide human genetic variations as results of interbreeding or mating between different populations previously isolated. These genetic variations observed in the human deoxyribonucleic acid (DNA) sequences are caused by inheritance processes, such as mutation and recombination. Generally, the mating process yields the genetic recombination break points, introduces some variations, and creates mixed DNA segments. As a consequence, current human populations are admixed [2, 3] with specific genomes displaying a mosaic of segments originating from different ancestral populations [1, 2, 4], wide phenotypic variations, divergent genetic ancestry, and different traits observed among individuals in worldwide population groups. Thus, it is critical to understand the dynamics related to the origin of these variations, the evolution process, and its consequences in human heredity and health.

Studying admixture patterns in human populations consists of characterization of admixture features in human populations, including admixture mapping and date to admixture events. Admixture mapping combines both the identification of genetic variants underlying the ethnic difference in disease risk and inference of ancestry estimates associated with these genetic variants. Estimation of ancestry is commonly known as genetic ancestry inference, which is either global or local ancestry inference. Global ancestry inference estimates the overall proportion contributed by each ancestral population to the admixed genome; while, local ancestry deconvolution (local ancestry inference) estimates the number of copies from a particular population at a given site [5]. Together, admixture mapping and date to admixture events provide a better understanding of the genetic variation features throughout modern human evolution, the demographics, and adaptive processes of human populations. Currently, analyzing admixture patterns has become central to genomics research, contributing to a wide range of biomedical applications. Current advance in technologies is facilitating the movement of people worldwide, thus influencing the complexity of population admixture dynamics and leading to multifaceted admixture events. On the other hand, the determination of local ancestry through genotyping and microarray datasets has empowered the approaches for dating mutation, selection, and admixture events [6, 7].

The significance of the local ancestry inference topic is viewed through the research interests it has raised over the last two decades. Several models exist for local ancestry deconvolution, including ANCESTRYMAP [8], ADMIXMAP [9], SABER [10], LAMP [11], LAMPLD/LAMPHAP [12], SUPPORTMIX [13], EILA [14], LOTER [15], etc. **Figure 1** displays the implementation dynamics of different local ancestry deconvolution models graphically, indicating the time each model was introduced. Local ancestry inference is relevant in personalizing medicines, understanding complex diseases, localizing missing sequences in reference genomes and understanding the population history and demographics. Subsequently, several studies have particularly been focusing on dating past admixture events, relevant to population migrations, heritable genes associated to some diseases, and responses to

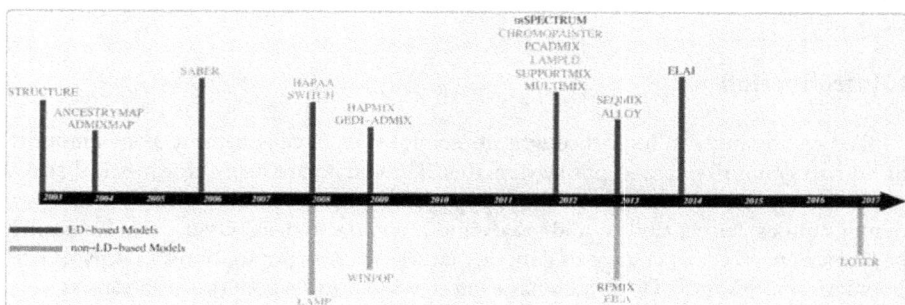

Figure 1.
The evolution of local ancestry deconvolution since 2003 to 2017.

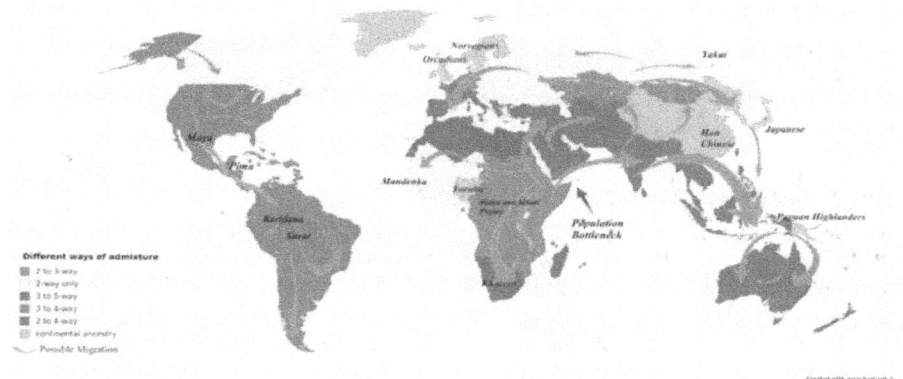

Figure 2.
A partial worldwide admixture painting map. The figure shows several worldwide admixed populations with patterns identified through published paper on population structure from 2008 to 2018. The population migrations within and between continents have resulted in different admixed populations ranging from one-to five-way admixtures.

treatment [16]. The date of admixture in a given population can be predicted by analyzing the ancestral track, break-points, and linkage disequilibrium (LD) [17]. Also, distinction between date of admixture events is made with the use of LD and ancestral tracts in the admixed genomes [17]. Nowadays, there are several models for predicting the age of an admixture event, which are classified into two main groups: LD-based approaches and haplotype-based approaches [17, 18]. These models use information from genomes of several population groups around the world as representative or equivalent ancient populations known to influence the migration and/or admixture processes, yielding observed admixed population patterns worldwide (**Figure 2**).

In this chapter, we survey current models for deconvoluting local ancestry and dating admixture events and explore computational techniques used in these models. We highlight advances made so far in this genomic era and opportunities behind these models and challenges or gaps that still need to be addressed. This informs users and researchers on the current state of research, and orient future trends in designing more effective models, which account for current challenges and produce more accurate and biological relevant estimates. In the subsequent sections, we provide an overview of existing methods used for inferring local ancestry estimates and dating admixture events.

2. Overview of admixture feature inference models

In this section, we survey current models used to elucidate admixture patterns, including local ancestry estimates (deconvolution) and dating admixture events. These models assume that the T genotyped sites are biallelic and the genotype information of the K reference candidate ancestral and admixed populations are considered known. Ancestry at different sites or windows follows a Markov chain. Recombination is assumed to occur at every generation resulting in Poison recombination points with a rate which depends on both the recombination rate, r, and number of generations since admixture, g, and individuals are independent of each other.

2.1 Local ancestry inference models

As pointed out previously, existing local ancestry inference models can be categorized into two main groups based on whether the model makes use of admixture/background linkage disequilibrium (LD) or not.

2.1.1 LD-based models for local ancestry inference

LD-based models account for LD in local ancestry deconvolution, and due to the importance of LD in disease mapping, the first local ancestry methods fall into this category. They assume that ancestry along an admixed individual genome follows a first order Markov chain. This means that the immediate past state captures all the information on past states [19]. As a result, LD-based models assume that, at every site, the observed admixed genotypes are generated by the unobserved ancestry, and hence, Hidden Markov Model (HMM) and its extensions are used to infer the unobserved (hidden) states. Thus, to deconvolute ancestry along the admixed genome, these models have three model parameters, namely the initial, transition and observation, or emission probability models. Due to uncertainty and the number of parameters involved, LD-based methods use Markov Chain Monte Carlo (MCMC), forward-backward, or Viterbi algorithms to determine the hidden ancestry sequence for a given individual. Falush et al. and Patterson et al. modeled ancestry switch between ancestry populations at a given site, $X_t \in \{1, ..., K\}$, by

$$P(X_1 = k|q, r) = q_k, \tag{1}$$

$$P\left(X_t = k|X_{t-1} = k', q, r\right) = \delta\left(k' = k\right)e^{-d_t r} + \left(1 - e^{-d_t r}\right)q_k \ \text{for} \ 1 < t \leq T \tag{2}$$

representing the first marker, and the transition probability between consecutive markers with $\delta\left(k = k'\right)$ is the indicator function and d_t the genetic distance between sites t and $t - 1$, above and q_k the proportion of ancestry contributed by candidate ancestral population k such that $q = (q_1, ..., q_k)$ is a vector of ancestry inherited from each ancestral population. On haploid data, the probability of a recombination event is $1 - e^{-d_t r}$, meaning that the probability of no recombination is $e^{-d_t r}$ [8, 20]. LD-based methods can be subdivided into admixture LD-based and admixture and background LD methods. Note that admixture LD occurs when ancestry at nearby markers is inherited together and background LD is the LD within ancestral populations, and it depends highly on population history (i.e, generated by genetic drift and population bottlenecks).

2.1.1.1 Admixture LD-based models

Admixture LD-based methods are models that account for LD that resulted from the admixture process. They do not model background LD. Admixture LD-based methods include the early methods, for example, STRUCTURE V2 [20], ANCESTRYMAP [8], and ADMIXMAP [9], which are based on the Bayesian framework. Early methods rely on markers that show significant difference in frequency between ancestral populations (AIMs). Admixture LD-based models assume that markers are independent and the global and ancestral allele frequencies are known. They integrate HMM with MCMC, and their switch model and initial and transition models are as in Eqs. (1) and (2), respectively. Since LD-based methods do not model background LD, their observation model depends on only the allele frequency of the ancestry at that site. For instance, assuming K = 2, Patterson et al. defined the emission probability by

$$P(Y_t = y | X_t = n_a) = \begin{cases} \begin{pmatrix} 2 \\ n_a \end{pmatrix} p_k^{n_a} (1 - p_k)^{2 - n_a} & if \ n_a = 0 \ or \ 1 \\ \begin{pmatrix} 2(1 - p_1)(1 - p_2) \\ p_2(1 - p_2) + p_1(1 - p_2) \\ p_1 p_2 \end{pmatrix} & if \ n_a = 2 \end{cases} \tag{3}$$

where y and $n_a \in \{0, 1\}$ are numbers of reference alleles of an admixed individual at t, and that of alleles from population 1, respectively. p_k is the allele frequency of population $k \in \{1, 2\}$ at the site t, such that when $n_a = 0$, $p_k = p_1$ while $p_k = p_2$ when $n_a = 2$. Nowadays, technological, statistical, and computational advances avail enormous amounts of high density SNP data. Although high density SNPs violate the independence assumption due to background LD [21], they contain more information than in AIMs [22]. To loosen the independence assumption and minimize noise and systematic biases from unmodelled LD, more advanced local ancestry inference methods emerged [22]. These methods include SEQMIX [23], PCADMIX [24], and SUPPORTMIX [13].

SUPPORTMIX [11] models only admixture LD by combining support vector machines (SVMs) and HMM. It was proposed in 2012 to improve on the computational time and address the challenge of a few typed or nonexistent reference panels, which overall improve multi-way local ancestry deconvolution. SUPPORTMIX is the first model to allow the learning of ancestral surrogates given a pool of reference panels. As a result, it is capable to train ancestral populations that are bigger in size than those that are mixed. Since SVMs can handle huge datasets, SUPPORTMIX is faster than early methods. It uses the rich haplotype information. Also proposed in 2012, PCADMIX [24] divides the genome into contiguous windows of SNPs as in SUPPORTMIX. It leverages principal component analysis from proxy ancestral haplotypes to model admixture LD under a standard HMM. Similar to SUPPORTMIX, PCADMIX is fast and requires phased data. Nevertheless, SUPPORTMIX and PCADMIX do not model phase switch errors, and as a result, in 2013, SEQMIX [23] was proposed. Unlike all other admixture LD-based methods, SEQMIX is based on exome sequence, reads data, and uses HMM. SEQMIX models only admixture LD and prunes SNPs in background LD. As a result, to reduce noise and systematic biases from using all SNPs [10] whilst not fully modeling LD (background), admixture and background LD methods emerged [22].

2.1.1.2 Admixture and background LD models

Since the biological data often have some dependences that violate the independence assumption in standard HMM, admixture LD-based methods are often not realistic. To relax the independence assumption, the HMM is extended to either Markov HMM, factorial HMM, hierarchical HMM, or two-layer HMM or other multivariate statistical models such as multivariate normal distribution (MVN) and a rich ancestral haplotype data are used unlike early methods. This is the case for SABER [10], SWITCH [25], HAPAA [26], HAPMIX [4], MULTIMIX [27], ALLOY [28], and ELAI [29]. MHMMs were the first HMM extension in local ancestry. They were first implemented in SABER and later in SWITCH. SABER was the first method to model background LD in the genetic ancestry inference. MHMM assumes that the current observed haplotype depends on both the current ancestry and the immediate past observation. The difference in the MHMM and admixture LD HMM-based is that when ancestry switches between sites t − 1 and t, then the MHMM observation model depends on the joint distribution of allele frequencies at the two sites [6, 30], defined as follows [10]:

$$P\left(Y_t = c | Y_{t-1} = d, X_t = k, X_{t'} = k'\right) = B_t\left(c, d, k', k\right),$$

$$P\left(Y_t = c | Y_{t-1} = d, X_t = k, X_{t'} = k'\right) = \begin{cases} \tilde{B}_{k',t}(c,d) \ \ for \ \ k' = k \\ \overline{B}_{k',t}(c) \ \ \ otherwise \end{cases} \tag{4}$$

where $\tilde{B}_{k,t}(c,d)$ is the probability of having alleles at marker t provided there was allele d at t − 1 and $\overline{B}_{k,t}(c)$ the allele frequency of alleles at marker t have for origins the population k. However, if the ancestry does not switch, then the observation model is like that of models in Section 2.1.1.1. The transition model of the SABER model accounts for the differences in admixture times that are in the real case of continuous gene flow where populations contribute their genetic material to the admixture in different generations [10]. Tang et al. defined the probability of switching from ancestry k at t to k at t as

$$A_{ij} = \begin{cases} q_i \dfrac{g_i^2}{\sum_{k=1}^{K} q_k g_k} - g_i, & for \ \ i = j, \\ q_j \dfrac{g_i g_j}{\sum_{k=1}^{K} q_k g_k}, & otherwise \end{cases} \tag{5}$$

where g_k is the admixture time when population k started to contribute to the admixture.

However, SABER has a large parameter set, and does not explicitly model background LD as it models background LD using first order Markov chain [22]; other methods such as SWITCH were proposed. SWITCH takes into recombination even if it does not result in an ancestry switch, emerged. In contrast to SABER, SWITCH conditions the MHMM on recombination. Similar to early methods, probability of recombination depends on the admixture generations, genetic distance between consecutive SNPs, and the recombination rate. Thus, if the transition probability model in SWITCH is marginalized over recombination, then it is similar to Eq. (2) for two-way and Eq. (5) for multi-way. Although SWITCH models background LD and estimates recombination rates, the authors recommended richer MHMM or other different models that would outperform the SWITCH and SABER pairwise models [25]. As a result, methods that use both large- and small-scale HMM, referred to as the HHMM, were introduced.

2.1.2 Non-LD-based local ancestry inference models

Non-LD methods neither model background nor admixture LD. They either remove SNPs in LD which is the case for LAMP [11] and WINPOP [31], or use all SNPs (linked and unlinked SNPs) without modeling LD; this is the case for EILA [14], RFMIX [32], and LOTER [15]. Since MHMMs have a large number of parameters and do not model LD explicitly, an algorithmic approach that divides genome into windows of SNPs, LAMP [11], emerged in 2008. LAMP is fast and robust, and can infer local ancestry even without proxy ancestral genotypes. This is the case for two-way admixtures. It uses the naive Bayes classifier and a clustering algorithm known as the iterative conditional modes. LAMP estimates the most probable ancestry at a site by applying the majority vote for each SNP [11]. Although accuracy is comprised, LAMP does not suffer from challenges of HMM and extension. As a result, LAMP underperforms in closely related populations, and hence it was extended to WINPOP [31], a dynamic programming algorithm. Unlike LAMP, WINPOP assumes at least one recombination event within each window and varies the window length depending on the genetic distance between populations. Hence, WINPOP and LAMP outperform other methods in closely and distantly related populations, respectively. Both LAMP and WINPOP assume unlinked markers and discards SNPs in LD.

As the admixed sequence data availability increases, Maples et al. proposed a discriminative approach to estimate local ancestry, RFMIX [32]. A discriminative approach estimates the posterior probability directly and not via the joint probability distribution. In contrast to generative ancestry inference models, RFMIX uses the information contained in admixed individuals. This is advantageous in cases of genotyped few reference panels. This is the case for Native Americans [32]. RFMIX uses conditional random fields (CRFs) parametrized on random forests. It outperforms in multi-way admixtures maybe due to modeling phase switch errors. In 2013, EILA [14], a multivariate statistic based method, was proposed particularly to increase inference power through addressing three common challenges in local ancestry. Addressed challenges are the independence of SNP assumption, difficulties in identifying break points, and the use of three genotype values. Instead of raw genotypes, EILA uses a numerical value between 0 and 1. The score determines how close SNPs are to the ancestral populations. Breakpoints are a challenge to identify, but EILA identifies them by fused quantile regression facilitating the use of estimates in admixture dating. Finally, k-means classifiers are used to infer ancestry using all genotyped SNPs [14].

Recently, a software package that deconvolves local ancestry in multi-way admixtures for a wide range of species, LOTER [15], was proposed. LOTER can account for phase errors in two-way admixture only. It facilitates the local ancestry inference process and its application in non-model species [15]. Unlike other methods, LOTER needs no biological such as admixture time and recombination rate or statistical parameters such as, number of hidden states and misfit probabilities to deconvolve ancestry [15]. Although it uses the Li and Stephen's copying model [33] as in LAMPLD/LAMPHAP, LOTER is a nonprobabilistic approach formulated from an optimization problem. Its solution is obtained through dynamic programming.

Finally, different existing LD and non-LD-based local ancestry inference models are summarized in **Table 1** extracted from Geza et al. [34].

2.2 Models for dating admixture events in a genome

Several models are now available to determine the date of admixture events in a given admixed genome. Breakpoints of haplotypes are used by some models while others focus on the ancestry blocks. Models based on ancestry blocks for dating admixture are formulated using either an empirical criteria or variants associated with a specific population. In order to determine the average length of the admixture block, these methods then assign ancestry on predefined windows using either wavelet transformation or conditional random fields [35]. On the other hand, there are models requiring rapid decrease in haplotype block sizes to estimate the date of the admixture event [36]. This suggests that, in general,

Software	Multi-way	Account LD	LD model	Biological/statistical parameters	Reference populations	Admixed populations	Year of publication
STRUCTURE V2*	✓	✓	HMM	Markers, and ancestry proportions	Unphased	Unphased	August 2003
ANCESTRYMAP*	✗	✓	HMM	Physical map, recombination and ancestry proportions	Unphased	Unphased	May 2004
ADMIXMAP*	✓	✓	HMM	Physical map and ancestry proportions	Unphased	Unphased	May 2004
SABER	✓	✓	MHMM	Physical map or recombination distance	Phased/unphased	Phased/unphased	July 2006
"LAMP"	✓	✗	✗	Admixture generations, LD threshold, and physical map	Unphased	Unphased	February 2008
HAPAA	✓	✓	HHMM	Admixture generations and genetic divergence	Phased	Phased	February 2008
SWITCH	✓	✓	MHMM	Recombination rate	Phased	Phased	February 2008
GEDI-ADMX	✓	✓	Fixed size FHMM	Admixed and ancestral SNPs (physical map)	Phased	Unphased	May 2009
WINPOP	✓	✗	✗	Recombination, admixture generations, LD threshold, and physical map	Unphased	Unphased	June 2009
HAPMIX	✗	✓	HHMM	Genetic map mutation rate and admixed and ancestral SNPs	Phased	Unphased	June 2009
CHROMOPAINTER	✓	✓	Co-ancestry matrix	Recombination rate	Phased	Phased	January 2012
LAMPLD	✓	✓	HHMM	Number of hidden states, window size and physical map	Phased	Unphased	May 2012
SUPPORTMIX*	✓	✓	HMM	Admixture generations and genetic map	Phased	Phased	June 2012
PCADMIX*	✓	✓	Windows of blocks of SNPs	Genetic map and window size	Phased	Phased	August 2012
mSPECTRUM	✓	✓		SNPs, mutation and recombination rate	Phased	Phased	August 2012
MULTIMIX	✓	✓	MVN	Genetic map, legend file and misfitting probabilities	Phased/unphased	Phased/unphased	November 2012

Software	Multi-way	Account LD	LD model	Biological/statistical parameters	Reference populations	Admixed populations	Year of publication
ALLOY	✓	✓	Non-homogeneous VLMC	Markers, ancestral proportions, admixture generations, and genetic map	Phased	Phased	February 2013
RFMIX	✓	✗	✗	Genetic map, window size, and admixture generations	Phased	Phased	August 2013
EILA	✓	✗	✗	Physical map	Unphased (no missing values)	Unphased (no missing values)	November 2013
SEQMIX	✓	✗	✗	Genetic map	Unphased	Unphased	November 2013
ELAI	✓	✓	Two layer HMM	Admixture generations, lower and upper cluster	Phased/unphased	Phased/unphased	May 2014
LOTER	✓	✗	✗	—	Phased	Phased	November 2017

Table 1.
Existing 20 ancestry deconvolution tools: ✓ indicates the ability of the software to perform a specified task, ✗ indicates the inapplicability of the task by a particular tool. Unless explicitly specified, LD refers to background LD.

models used for dating admixture events can be subdivided in two main classes [17, 18], namely those based on LD and those based on the haplotype distribution, as mentioned earlier.

2.2.1 LD-based models for dating admixture events

An admixture event is mainly characterized by the transfer of genes from the ancestral populations to the admixed ones. This leads to the appearance of linkage disequilibrium with regard to the ancestral populations. However, this LD formed often decreases with time. Also, the rate of decay of LD is a function of recombination and the proportion of the admixture [35]. Inversely, many methods employ this rate to calculate the time since the admixture event occurs.

In 2011, Moorjani et al. introduced a method to determine the weighted correlation for a pair of SNPs [36]. This correlation coefficient is further used to measure the LD with ancestral populations [37]. The time of admixture is then determined by analyzing the correlation with respect to the genetic distance, and also fitting using a least squares method the decay of the correlation [35]. This method got improved in 2011 by Loh et al. [18]. The major improvements are in terms of computation. Loh et al. employed instead a fast Fourier transform and other faster techniques to determine the optimal distance to the fitting curve. This method has another advantage that it reduces considerable biases in the estimation of the time of admixture [18, 36]. Later, Loh et al.'s method was improved by Pickrell et al. [38] by introducing the notion of mixture exponential decay in order to take into account the admixture events in the given admixed population history. It mainly focuses on the decay of the LD.

2.2.1.1 Multiple weighted correlation coefficient

Let us consider three ancestral populations k_1, k_2, and k_3, and Q the admixed population. Let us denote by ω_{1-2}, ω_{1-3}, and ω_{2-3} three weighted linkage disequilibrium scores computed based on all possible pairs of SNPs between the three ancestral populations: $k_1 - k_2$, $k_1 - k_3$, and $k_2 - k_3$, respectively, in the admixed population Q calculated using the method proposed by Loh et al. According to Prickrell et al., the multiple weighted correlation coefficient is [38],

$$C_{k_1-k_2, k_1-k_2, k_2-k_3} = \sqrt{\frac{\omega_{2-3}^2 + \omega_1^2 - 2\omega_{2-3}\omega_{1-2}\omega_{1-3}}{1 - \omega_{2-3}^2}}. \tag{6}$$

The date of admixture between population k_1 and k_3 is

$$D_{k_1, k_2, k_1 k_2 - k_2 k_3} = \begin{cases} w_0 + w_1 e^{-n_1 \frac{\delta_n}{100}}, & \text{for one admixture event} - D_{(1)}, \\ w_0 + w_1 e^{-n_1 \frac{\delta_n}{100}} + w_2 e^{-n_2 \frac{\delta_n}{100}}, & \text{in the case of two admixture events} - D_{(2)}, \end{cases} \tag{7}$$

with n_1 and n_1 the number of generations; δ_n the genetic distance; w_1 and w_2 stand for the value of the multiple weighted LD; and w_0 the affine term. $D_{(1)}$ is the date of admixture of population Q in the case of admixture either between $k_1 - k_2$ or $k_2 - k_3$. On the other hand, if it is assumed that two admixture events took place between $k_1 - k_3$ and either $k_1 - k_2$ or $k_2 - k_3$, the date of the admixed population is given by $D_{(2)}$.

2.2.2 Haplotype distribution-based models for dating admixture events

Among the haplotype-based approaches, there is the likelihood method introduced in 2009 by Price et al. [4]. It basically determines the number of breakpoints using Hidden Markov Model. It is also able to determine the number of alleles at a particular site inherited from a given ancestor in a population. This is done in two steps. First, the method consists in identifying haplotype from the proxy ancestry populations, and secondly, the origin of each haplotype bock is identified by comparing their likelihood for one ancestral population versus the others. Considering an admixed genome, the likelihood of an observed allele is given by

$$H_{uvw}(h) = \begin{cases} \theta_u P(t_{vw} = 0) + (1 - \theta_u)P(t_{vw} = 1), \text{ if } u = v, \\ \theta_3 P(t_{vw} = 0) + (1 - \theta_3)P(t_{vw} = 1), \quad \text{otherwise} \end{cases} \tag{8}$$

with θ_u, $u \in \{1, 2, 3\}$ the mutation parameter is; h represents the haplotype site in the chromosomal offspring; the function t_{vw} is an indicator function. It takes the value 1 if individual w coming from offspring x has the same haplotype with the ancestral population v and 0 otherwise; and P is the probability to inherit a pair of haplotype [4]. The number of generations since admixture is given by

$$G = \frac{C}{4\gamma(1 - \gamma)\zeta} \tag{9}$$

where ζ is the total Morgan length, γ the proportion of admixture, and C the observed number of breakpoints [4].

On the other hand, Pugach et al. [17] employed the wavelet transform to design a haplotype block approach. The aim of this method is to derive the time of admixture of a given population using the simple hybrid isolation model. It proceeds in two main steps. First, it obtains a signal of admixture from the admixed data using the principal component technique. The second step consists in deriving the date of admixture using the signal obtained in the first step [17].

Pool and Nielsen also built a haplotype-based approach. It used precautionary ancestral populations to infer the date of admixture from the genome of an admixed population [39]. It assumed that after a number of generation g, the distribution of the ancestral haplotypes follows exponential distribution given by

$$f(\lambda, g) = ge^{-\lambda g} \tag{10}$$

where λ is the length of haplotypes. Also, the mean of this distribution is known and is equal to $\frac{1}{g}$.

Further methods include that of Gravel developed in 2012 for the identification of multiple ancestral populations in a given admixture dataset [40]. Also, Jin et al. [41] came up with a similar method to explain admixture dynamics. The method incorporates several models including gradual admixture (GA), hybrid isolated (HI), and continuous gene flow (CGF) models [41], which can be extended to GA-Isolation (GA-I) and CGF-Isolation (CGF-I) by considering isolation after admixture [42]. Hellenthal et al. [43] on the other hand built up on the work of Lawson et al. [44] on dating admixture. This method particularly considers the genome of an admixed individual to be a set chunk DNA coming from other individuals. The scheme of this method is mainly made of two stages. The first stage consists in dividing the genome into chunks and matching each of them to the proper ancestral individual. This stage is achieved with the help of Hidden Markov

Model. The second stage consists in identifying haplotypes and determining their respective ancestral population [43, 44]. Moreover, the admixture event and its date are derived by fitting the decay of the ancestral haplotype with an exponential distribution curve. Moreover, Ni et al. developed a method based on the observation that the date of admixture events is related to the model used. Their method consists in using the likelihood ratio test to identify the best model for the inference of the date of admixture. Furthermore, they are able to estimate several admixture events with the given optimal model [35].

Finally, different existing models and tools for dating admixture events are summarized in **Table 2** extracted from Chimusa et al. [35].

Tool	Category	Admixture model	Priori proxy ancestral raw data	Multi-way events	Online link
ROLLOFF	LD-based model	HI	Yes	No	https://github.com/DReichLab/AdmixTools/
ALDER		HI	Yes	No	http://cb.csail.mit.edu/cb/alder/
MALDER		HI	Yes	Yes	https://github.com/joepickrell/malder/
CAMer		HI, GA, CGF, GA-I, CGF-I	Yes	Yes	https://github.com/david940408/CAMer
IMAAPs		HI, GA, CGF, GA-I, CGF-I	Yes	Yes	http://www.picb.ac.cn/PGG/resource.php
StepPCO	Haplotype/ ancestry block size distribution-based model	HI	Yes	Yes	https://bioinf.eva.mpg.de/download/StepPCO/
Adware		HI, Dual-admixture	Yes	Yes	https://cran.r-project.org/web/packages/adwave/index.html
HAPMIX		HI	Yes	Yes	http://genetics.med.harvard.edu/reichlab/Reich_Lab/Software.html/
MultiWaveIner		HI	Yes	Yes	https://github.com/xyang619/MultiWaveInfer/ or http://www.picb.ac.cn/PGG/resource.php
GLOBBERTROTTER		HI, GA, CGF	No	Yes	https://github.com/maarjalepamets/human-admixture/
Tracts		HI, GA, CGF	No	Yes	https://github.com/sgravel/tracts/
Ancestry_HMM		HI	No	No	https://github.com/russcd/

Table 2.
Existing dating admixture genomic tools.

3. Challenges and perspectives

3.1 Case of local ancestry inference models

Although several models exist to deconvolve local ancestry, most studies that evaluate such models showed that deviations in local ancestry estimates still exist in multi-way admixtures. Deviations in local ancestry also result from genetic drift, miscalling true ancestry, and genotyping errors. However, the signals from these factors affect the whole genome while that of unmodelled natural selection affects particular regions. For example, Chen et al. using four local ancestry inference models to scan for disease-related loci through admixture mapping showed that although all of them are LD based and divide the genome into windows of continuous SNPs, MULTIMIX and LAMPLD estimates differed in almost 20% of the analyzed SNPs. This results from the differences in the biological and statistical parameters they require and the mathematical approaches they use. Another association study by Chimusa et al. [45] also pointed out that admixture mapping is still limited by inaccuracies in multi-way local ancestry deconvolution when they evaluated one LD-based and one non-LD-based local ancestry models, WINPOP and LAMPLD.

Inaccuracies in local ancestry estimates may result from the use of statistical or biological parameters in the estimation process, which are not always accurate when provided. It could also be due to the dependence of models on reference panels which for some populations are few or even not sampled for others. This is the case for the Native Americans. More so for other admixed populations, their history is not well known. When applied to ancient admixtures, existing methods may yield spurious estimates as they were designed for recent admixtures. Existing methods do not account for natural selection; hence, some deviations exist in regions that are under selection [45]. Also, most of them are benchmarked for three-way admixtures.

Since each model was introduced to address a particular challenge that models before it faced, it is clearly expected that no model or tool can achieve the best performance in all admixture scenarios and not trading estimate accuracy with computational speed. Using existing studies by Geza et al. [34], more than 50% of studies that either introduced a model or evaluated methods for association mapping showed that LAMPLD/LAMPHAP outperforms most LD-based methods. And the only LD-based method than outperformed LAMPLD is ELAI; however, this is the only study that assessed ELAI with other models. In cases where LD-based models were compared to non-LD-based models, RFMIX outperformed LAMPLD in three cases highlighted in [34], while another separate study aiming to determine the place of admixture of an admixed population RFMIX also outperformed. This could be because RFMIX can deconvolve ancestry in closely related populations [46]. However, a recent assessment between RFMIX and LOTER resulted in LOTER outperforming in ancient admixtures [15].

Generally, each model is implemented as a tool in local ancestry deconvolution, existing as individual scripts requiring unique inputs and producing unique outputs. This challenges researchers with a limited computational background; thus, there is lack of a unified framework which can require a standard easy to manipulate input files and output results in a way that is easy to process for further application. In conclusion, for informed decisions on models and algorithms, existing models or tools should be assessed within a unified framework. This will allow them to be tested on different admixture scenarios and also incorporating most state-of-the-art LD and non-LD based models.

3.2 Case of the dating admixture models

The evolution of human populations and the history of the mixture of these populations have been deciphered using statistical and computational methods. These methods have been found to perform well when dealing with single point admixture event in two-way admixed populations [35]. However, as any method, they not only have advantages but also pitfalls regarding the estimation of admixture dates in some cases. It is challenging to fit to real admixed populations (for more than 3-way admixture context) in the existing models dating admixture events due to several reasons, including reliance to optimal local ancestry estimates and accurate ancestry breakpoints. This suggests that there is still a need for designing an integrative or a new model to dating admixture events for current multi-way admixed populations to further advance our understanding of human demographics and movement, and facilitate admixture mapping and estimation of the age of a disease locus contributing to disease risk.

In addition, it have been discovered that the mixture exponential decay model over-estimates the date of older admixture events [35] and was suggested to detect at most three admixture events. As mentioned earlier, Ni et al. [47] dealt with the optimization of the method used in dating admixture estimation. They took into account several models but the evaluation of their technique is not effective in the estimation of ancient and multi admixture events [35, 47]. On the other hand, several practical considerations can further limit these approaches including the use of proxy ancestry populations in the estimations which could bias the accuracy of the result. This is the case when dealing for instance with low sample size and inappropriate proxy ancestral populations [35]; the requirement of having accurate LD patterns, ancestry haplotypes distribution, and a big sample size of the admixed population. Thus, there is a need for an adequate model for inferring different dates of admixture events and matching real admixture history using proxy ancestry-based methods [35].

4. Conclusions

Currently, more than 20 models exist and are implemented as software to deconvolve local ancestry and 12 tools for dating admixture events. In this chapter, we discussed in detail and summarized the most commonly used models, the model assumptions, statistical and biological parameters they require, and existing challenges. This discussion highlights the need for designing more effective models, which account for current challenges and produce more accurate and biologically relevant estimates. Furthermore, it provides useful information for the implementation of practical tools, which consider current medical and population genetic demands. More importantly, this may guide users in the choice of appropriate tools for specific applications and can assist software developers in designing more advanced tools for local ancestry deconvolution and dating admixture events.

Acknowledgements

Some of the authors are supported in part by the National Institutes of Health (NIH) Common Fund [grant numbers U24HG006941 (H3ABioNet) and 1U01HG007459–01 (SADaCC)]. One of the authors is fully funded by the Organization for Women in Science for the Developing World (OWSD) and Swedish International Development Cooperation Agency (Sida). The content of this publication is solely the responsibility of the authors and does not necessarily represent the official views of the funders.

Conflict of interest

The authors declare that they have no competing interest.

Author details

Gaston K. Mazandu[1,2,3*], Ephifania Geza[1,3], Milaine Seuneu[1,2] and Emile R. Chimusa[2]

1 African Institute for Mathematical Sciences (AIMS), Cape Town, South Africa

2 Division of Human Genetics, Department of Pathology, Faculty of Health Sciences, Institute of Infectious Disease and Molecular Medicine, University of Cape Town (UCT), Cape Town, South Africa

3 Computational Biology Division, Department of Integrative Biomedical Sciences, University of Cape Town, South Africa

*Address all correspondence to: kuzamunu@aims.ac.za

IntechOpen

References

[1] Cavalli-Sforza LL, Feldman MW. The application of molecular genetic approaches to the study of human evolution. Nature Genetics. 2003;**33**: 266-275

[2] A. Koehl, Estimating Ancestry and Genetic Diversity in Admixed Populations. The University of New Mexico. Thesis 2016

[3] Yang JJ, Cheng C, Devidas M, Cao X, Fan Y, Campana D, et al. Ancestry and pharmacogenomics of relapse in acute lymphoblastic leukemia. Nature Genetics. 2011;**43**(3):237-241

[4] Price AL, Tandon A, Patterson N, Barnes KC, Rafaels N, Ruczinski I, et al. Sensitive detection of chromosomal segments of distinct ancestry in admixed populations. PLoS Genetics. 2009;**5**(6):e1000519

[5] Thornton TA, Bermejo JL. Local and global ancestry inference and applications to genetic association analysis for admixed populations. Genetic Epidemiology. 2014;**38**(S1): S5-S12

[6] Liu Y, Nyunoya T, Leng S, et al. Softwares and methods for estimating genetic ancestry in human populations. Human Genomics. 2013;**7**(1):1

[7] Bhatia G, Patterson N, Pasaniuc B, et al. Genome-wide comparison of African-ancestry populations from care and other cohorts reveals signals of natural selection. American Journal of Human Genetics. 2011;**89**: 368-381

[8] Patterson N, Hattangadi N, Lane B, Lohmueller KE, Hafler DA, Oksenberg JR, et al. Methods for high-density admixture mapping of diseases genes. The American Journal of Human Genetics. 2004;**74**(5):979-1000

[9] Hoggart CJ, Shriver MD, Kittles RA, Clayton DG, McKeigue PM. Design and analysis of admixture mapping studies. The American Journal of Human Genetics. 2004;**74**(5):965-978

[10] Tang H, Coram M, Wang P, Zhu X, Risch N. Reconstructing genetic ancestry blocks in admixed individuals. The American Journal of Human Genetics. 2006;**79**(1):1-12

[11] Sankararaman S, Sridhar S, Kimmel G, Halperin E. Estimating local ancestry in admixed populations. The American Journal of Human Genetics. 2008;**82**(2): 290-303

[12] Baran Y, Pasaniuc B, Sankararaman S, Torgerson DG, Gignoux C, Eng C, et al. Fast and accurate inference of local ancestry in latino populations. Bioinformatics. 2012;**28**(10):1359-1367

[13] Omberg L, Salit J, Hackett N, Fuller J, Matthew R, Chouchane L, et al. Inferring genome-wide patterns of admixture in qataris using fifty-five ancestral populations. BMC Genetics. 2012;**13**(1):49

[14] Yang JJ, Li J, Buu A, Williams LK. Efficient enference of local ancestry. Bioinformatics. 2013;**29**(21):2750-2756

[15] Dias-Alves T, Mairal J, Blum MG. Loter: A software package to infer local ancestry for a wide range of species. Molecular Biology and Evolution. 2018; **35**(7):msy126

[16] Cheng R, Lim J, Samocha K, et al. Genome-wide association studies and the problem of relatedness among advanced intercross lines and other highly recombinant populations. Genetics. 2010;**185**:1033-1044

[17] Pugach I, Matveyev R, Wollstein A, et al. Dating the age of admixture via

wavelet transform analysis of genome-wide data. Genome Biology. 2011;**12**:R19

[18] Loh P-R, Lipson M, Patterson N, et al. Inferring admixture histories of human populations using linkage disequilibrium. Genetics. 2013;**193**: 1233-1254

[19] Murphy KP. Machine Learning: A Probabilistic Perspective. Cambridge, Massachusetts, London: MIT press; 2012

[20] Falush D, Stephens M, Pritchard JK. Inference of population structure using multilocus genotype data: Linked loci and correlated allele frequencies. Genetics. 2003;**164**(4):1567-1587

[21] Chen X, Ishwaran H. Random forests for genomic data analysis. Genomics. 2012;**99**(6):323-329

[22] Seldin MF, Pasaniuc B, Price AL. New approaches to disease mapping in admixed populations. Nature Reviews Genetics. 2011;**12**(8):523-528

[23] Hu Y, Willer C, Zhan X, Kang HM, Abecasis G. Accurate local-ancestry inference in exome-sequenced admixed individuals via off-target sequence reads. The American Journal of Human Genetics. 2013;**93**(5):891-899

[24] Brisbin A, Bryc K, Byrnes J, Zakharia F, Omberg L, Degenhardt J, et al. PCAdmix: Principal components-based assignment of ancestry along each chromosome in individuals with admixed ancestry from two or more populations. Human Biology. 2012; **84**(4):343

[25] Sankararaman S, Kimmel G, Halperin E, Jordan MI. On the inference of ancestries in admixed populations. Genome Research. 2008;**18**(4):668-675

[26] Sundquist A, Fratkin E, Do CB, Batzoglou S. Effect of genetic divergence in identifying ancestral

origin using HAPAA. Genome Research. 2008;**18**(4):676-682

[27] Churchhouse C, Marchini J. Multiway admixture deconvolution using phased or unphased ancestral panels. Genetic Epidemiology. 2013; **37**(1):1-12

[28] Rodriguez JM, Bercovici S, Elmore M, Batzoglou S. Ancestry inference in complex admixtures via variable-length Markov chain linkage models. Journal of Computational Biology. 2013;**20**(3): 199-211

[29] Guan Y. Detecting structure of haplotypes and local ancestry. Genetics. 2014;**196**(3):625-642

[30] Padhukasahasram B. Inferring ancestry from population genomic data and its applications. Frontiers in Genetics.5:204

[31] Paşaniuc B, Sankararaman S, Kimmel G, Halperin E. Inference of locus-specific ancestry in closely related populations. Bioinformatics. 2009; **25**(12):i213-i221

[32] Maples BK, Gravel S, Kenny EE, Bustamante CD. RFMix: A discriminative modeling approach for rapid and robust local-ancestry inference. The American Journal of Human Genetics. 2013;**93**(2): 278-288

[33] Li N, Stephens M. Modeling linkage disequilibrium and identifying recombination hotspots using single-nucleotide polymorphism data. Genetics. 2003;**165**(4):2213-2233

[34] Geza E, Mugo J, Mulder NJ, Wonkam A, Chimusa ER, Mazandu GK. A comprehensive survey of models for dissecting local ancestry deconvolution in human genome. Briefings in Bioinformatics. 2018. DOI: 10.1093/bib/bby044

[35] Chimusa ER, Defo J, Thami PK, Awany D, Mulisa DD, Allali I, et al. Dating admixture events is unsolved problem in multi-way admixed populations. Briefings in Bioinformatics. 2018:1-58. https://doi.org/10.1093/bib/bby112

[36] Moorjani P, Thangaraj K, Patterson N, et al. Genetic evidence for recent population mixture in India. Human Genetics. 2013;**93**:422-438

[37] Moorjani P, Patterson N, Hirschhorn J, et al. The history of African gene flow into Southern Europeans, Levantines, and Jews. PLoS Genetics. 2011;7:e1001373

[38] Pickrell J, Reich D. Toward a new history and geography of human genes informed by ancient DNA. Trends in Genetics. 2014;**30**:377-389

[39] Pool J, Nielsen R. Inference of historical changes in migration rate from the lengths of migrant tracts. Genetics. 2009;**181**:711-719

[40] Gravel S. Population genetics models of local ancestry. Genetics. 2012; **191**:607-619

[41] Jin W, Li R, Zhou Y, et al. Distribution of ancestral chromosomal segments in admixed genomes and its implications for inferring population history and admixture mapping. Human Genetics. 2014;**22**:930

[42] Zhou Y, Qiu H, Xu S. Modeling continuous admixture using admixture-induced linkage disequilibrium. Scientific Reports. 2017;7:43054

[43] Hellenthal G, Busby G, Band G, et al. A genetic atlas of human admixture history. Science. 2014;**434**: 747-751

[44] Lawson D, Hellenthal G, Myers S, et al. Inference of population structure using dense haplotype data. PLoS Genetics. 2012;**8**:e1002453

[45] Chimusa ER, Zaitlen N, Daya M, Møller M, van Helden PD, Mulder NJ, et al. Genome-wide association study of ancestry-specific tb risk in the South African coloured population. Human Molecular Genetics. 2014;**23**(3):796-809

[46] Xue J, Lencz T, Darvasi A, Pe'er I, Carmi S. The time and place of European admixture in Ashkenazi Jewish history. PLoS Genetics. 2017; **13**(4):e1006644

[47] Ni X, Yuan K, Yang X, et al. Inference of multiple-wave admixtures by length distribution of ancestral tracks. Heredity (Edinb). 2018;**121**:52-63

Recognition of Multiomics-Based Molecule-Pattern Biomarker for Precise Prediction, Diagnosis, and Prognostic Assessment in Cancer

Xanquan Zhan, Tian Zhou, Tingting Cheng and Miaolong Lu

Abstract

Cancer is a complex whole-body chronic disease, is involved in multiple causes, multiple processes, and multiple consequences, which are associated with a series of molecular alterations in the different levels of genome, transcriptome, proteome, metabolome, and radiome, with between-molecule mutual interactions. Those molecule-panels are the important resources to recognize the reliable molecular pattern biomarkers for precise prediction, diagnosis, and prognostic assessment in cancer. Pattern recognition is an effective methodology to identify those molecule-panels. The rapid development of computation biology, systems biology, and multiomics is driving the development of pattern recognition to discover reliable molecular pattern biomarkers for cancer treatment. This book chapter addresses the concept of pattern recognition and pattern biomarkers, status of multiomics-based molecular patterns, and future perspective in prediction, diagnosis, and prognostic assessment of a cancer.

Keywords: cancer, multiomics, genomics, transcriptomics, proteomics, metabolomics, radiomics, molecule-pattern biomarker, pattern recognition

1. Introduction

Cancer is a leading cause of death worldwide, with increasing morbidity and mortality. Studies indicated that the number of new cancer case per year will be 19.3 million by 2025, and more than half of cancer cases and mortality occur in developing countries and the proportion tendency is estimated to increase by 2025 [1]. Cancer is a complex process involving multiple causes, multiple processes, and multiple consequences, which are associated with a series of molecular alterations in the different levels of genome, transcriptome, proteome, metabolome, and radiome, with between-molecule mutual interactions. Cancer arises when normal cells' orderly processes controlled multiplication and life span were interfered. It is also reported that person's genetic makeup and lifestyle factors such as diet, alcohol, smoke, and physical activity, influence the rate at which cancer develops and progresses.

Alterations or mutations of genetic substance of the cells are the main cause of changes in cellular behavior. Dysregulation of the normal cellular procedure in cancer for cell fission, differentiation, apoptosis and proliferation is due to alterations in multiple genes expression and leading to an imbalance between cell replication and cell death, which is beneficial for growth of tumor cell population [2, 3]. With cancer progresses, the genetic drift of the cell population generates cell heterogeneity with characteristics involved in cell antigenicity, invasiveness, metastatic potential, rate of cell proliferation, differentiation state and response to chemotherapeutic agents [4–6]. A study showed that the mutation of two to eight driver genes is sufficient for an emblematical cancer occurrence. The passenger genes are not oncogenic and mutation of passenger genes is unable to cause occurrence of a cancer [7, 8]. Therefore, attention should be paid to a panel of genetic mutations, named gene pattern mutation. Depending on the genetic central dogma, gene pattern mutation may lead to a series of alterations of messenger RNA (mRNA) and protein expressions. With the use of this pattern, the condition of low sensitivity of a single-tumor marker or low specificity of a large number of samples is reduced when diagnosis models are set based on differentially expressed proteins or peptides between tumor tissues and normal tissues [9].

A cancer biomarker is defined as a substance or biological process that can indicate the presence of cancer in the body, which is important for people to monitor personal health [10]. Physical examinations (e.g., blood pressure), biological and genetic tests, along with others that can be objectively detected and used as indicators of pathogenic processes and alterations which may present as a result of treatment, are regarded as biomarkers [11, 12]. All the alterations in the levels of DNA, RNA, protein, and metabolite between cancer patients and healthy people could be called biomarkers, and therefore in terms of source, biomarkers usually are assorted into different categories including genetic biomarker, epigenetic biomarker, protein biomarker, metabolite biomarker and immunological biomarker and so on [13]. Generally, biomarkers used in clinic survey and diagnosis are from the four ways: (i) metabolites of tumor cells, (ii) abnormal differentiation of cellular gene products, (iii) tumor necrosis and exfoliation of tumor cells release into the blood circulation, and (iv) cell reactive products of tumor host cells [9]. Most of cancer biomarkers are detected in the tumor tissue or in blood. In order to maximize usefulness and minimize cost of screening or early detection, it is advantageous to be able to measure biomarkers in body fluid, which can be obtained using minimally invasive samples, such as blood, urine, sputum or stool [10]. Biomarkers play an important role in cancer for precise prediction, diagnosis and prognostic assessment. Thereby, with the development of biomarkers, they have far-reaching significances for people to recognize and treat cancer as follows: (i) the understanding of molecular mechanisms of diseases, (ii) identification of possible new disease pathways, (iii) prediction models of complex diseases, (iv) the determination of the level of biological activity of the disease, (v) refinement of disease phenotypes that may respond differently to specific treatments, (vi) the monitoring of treatment responses, and (vii) the potential application of precision medicine [14, 15]. However, it still remains a problem that biomarkers were detected after occurrence of cancer. With the fast development of image technology, radiomics is generated and can well solve that above problem. Quantitative analysis of imaging characteristics provides not only the tumor phenotype but also the underlying genotype information so that one can better diagnose and prognostic assessment for cancer patients [16]. A single tumor biomarker is insufficient and unreliable for precise prediction, diagnosis and prognostic assessment in cancer. The multi-parameter systematic strategies for predictive, preventive, and personalized medicine (PPPM) in cancer [4] emphasized that those molecule-panels, all of the differences and molecular alterations in the genome, transcriptome, proteome, metabolome, and radiome, with between-molecule mutual interactions, are the important resources to identify and recognize the reliable molecular pattern biomarkers for precise prediction, diagnosis, and prognostic assessment in cancer. Pattern recognition is an effective methodology to identify those molecule-panels. In fact, pattern recognition means that recognize molecule-pattern biomarkers, in other words, to use a set of patterns that consist of several biomarkers to improve the accuracy and specificity of prediction, prevention, diagnosis, treatment, and prognostic assessment of tumor [9].

The rapid development of computation biology, systems biology, and multiomics is driving the development of pattern recognition to discover reliable molecular pattern biomarkers for cancer treatment. This book chapter addresses the concept of pattern recognition and pattern biomarkers, status of multiomics-based molecular patterns, and future perspective in prediction, diagnosis, and prognostic assessment of a cancer.

2. Pathophysiological basis of molecule-pattern biomarker in cancer

Cancer is a complex whole-body chronic disease, which results in a series of molecular alterations and associated with signal transduction system, cell cycle, proliferation, differentiation and apoptosis [17, 18]. Many factors are related to occurrence and development of a cancer.

Genomic instability plays a key role in cancer development and progression. It provides a way to make a cell or subset of cells gain an ability of selective advantage than adjacent cells, achieving outgrowth and advantages in the tissue microenvironment. Genomic instability can generate aneuploid cells. Aneuploidy influences on the transcriptome and proteome and further results in proteotoxic stress and activation of the endoplasmic reticulum stress response. Consequently, aneuploidy can regulate features of the cells and the microenvironment [19]. In normal cells, the quality of reproduction of the genome at each stage of the cell cycle is protected by checkpoints. The existence of aneuploid cells in cancer exactly suggested one or more checkpoints are failed. The genomic heterogeneity might provide growth advantages for cancer "tissue" under selection pressure, such as hypoxia, immunity, and treatment-related challenges [1]. Genomic instability in cancer causes a serious challenge for cancer treatment.

Genetic mutations that cause cell dysfunction in most of cases support the development and progression of cancer. Moreover, the interaction between cancer cells and their environment, known as the tumor microenvironment, and their mutually interacted regulatory factors, can affect disease initiation and progression. The tumor microenvironment is composed of stromal cells, extracellular matrix (ECM), and signaling molecules that communicate with cancer cells. The stromal cells including endothelial cells, pericytes, fibroblasts, and immune cells, along with the surrounding ECM, constitute a supporting matrix for the tumor and regulate the tumor microenvironment. Angiogenesis and metastasis, two pivotal hallmarks of cancer, are modulated by the composition of the tumor microenvironment. Furthermore, the tumor microenvironment is not only affected by signals from tumor cells, but also stromal components through influencing cancer cell function to promote tumor progression and metastasis [20, 21]. Therefore, tumor microenvironment also is an important aspect for cancer therapy.

Tumor heterogeneity is another momentous feature of malignant tumor and plays a vital role in development, progression, and treatment of cancer [22–26]. On the one hand, in most of cancer cases, heterogeneity is found that not only from same kind of tumor among different patients, but also in all tumor progression phases of the identical individual patients [27]. The genetic instability of tumor cell is tightly related to tumor progression and heterogeneity and leads to the presence of variations [28, 29]. On the other hand, tumor heterogeneity is relevant to the individual differences between tumor patients. For example, the function of liver and kidney, age, physical condition, psychological status and personal lifestyle factors, are also another important factors which affect on the tumor progression and treatment [30]. A number of treatment plans of patients were designed according to the doctor's experiences and adopted same therapy model for different cancer patients in clinic. Due to ignore tumor heterogeneity, the "one-size-fits-all" therapeutic model resulted in the expected curative effect could not completely be achieved [4]. Thereby, tumor heterogeneity is becoming an important factor to hinder the effective treatment and cancer research.

Molecular mechanisms of initiation and progression of a cancer do not just exist one kind of intracellular signal pathway [31]. Several researches have indicated that phosphoinositide 3-kinase/protein kinase B (PI3K/Akt), mitogen-activated protein kinase (MAPK) and signal transducer, and activator of transcription 3 (STAT3) pathways were activated in obesity-associated colon cancer. Mammalian target of rapamycin (mTOR) as a down-stream of both PI3K/Akt and MAPK is highly activated [32]. Activated mTOR in proper order inhibits the PI3K/Akt pathway and further activates the STAT3 pathway [33]. In case that mTOR is inhibited, the activity of PI3K/Akt may obviously increase owing to the feedback inhibition of mTOR on PI3K activity [34]. Therefore, it is necessary to simultaneously suppress the expressions of mTOR and PI3K for the treatment of obesity-related cancer [4]. Hence one can see that the interaction and interrelationship of multiple signaling pathways is essential to pay more attention to study, and a single signaling molecule or biomarker is unreliable for the prediction, diagnosis, and treatment of cancer.

So far, there are many kinds of treatments for cancer including surgery, radiotherapy, and systemic treatments including cytotoxic chemotherapy, hormonal therapy, immunotherapy, and targeted therapies [35]. Personalized or individualized variations are related to human healthcare, and the relationship is shown (**Figure 1**). Three primary stages, prediction/prevention, early-stage diagnosis/ early-stage therapy, and late-stage diagnosis/late-stage therapy are involved in human healthcare. Personalized or individualized variations can be used as biomarkers for prediction, and further the assessment of preventive response reflects the results of preventive treatments. Personalized or individualized variations also can be regarded as diagnostic biomarkers and further for cancer therapy. The assessment of therapeutic response, known as prognostic assessment, consists in early-stage therapy and late-stage therapy, and reveals the influence of therapeutic intervention. Of the three stages, prediction/prevention is the most significant part due to make people keep on a healthy condition and be treated in time once cancer occurs. Early-stage diagnosis/therapy also is better approach to block and repress the progression of cancer while the preventive strategy failed. Late-stage diagnosis/therapy is also named clinical diagnosis and treatment of a cancer. Unluckily, most of cancer cases were found in late stage. In order to avoid aforementioned problem and improve people's health level, many researchers concentrate on exploration of biomarkers on prediction/prevention and early-stage diagnosis/therapy for cancer [4]. According to functional classification, biomarkers are divided into two categories (**Table 1**): (i) serving for the mechanism and therapeutic targets, and (ii) devoting to prediction, diagnostic test, and prognosis assessment. The first kind of biomarkers is relevant to the initiation and development of disease, and directly indicates the mechanism and pathogenesis of the disease. Commonly, it is pivotal site in cell signal pathways, like P53 in nasopharyngeal carcinoma (NPC) [36]. Another kind of biomarkers does not need to be causal to the occurrence and development of the disease, but requires to be provided with specificity and a certain number of changes to be easily detected. Based on Bayes' rule, three or more key molecules can form molecule-pattern biomarker

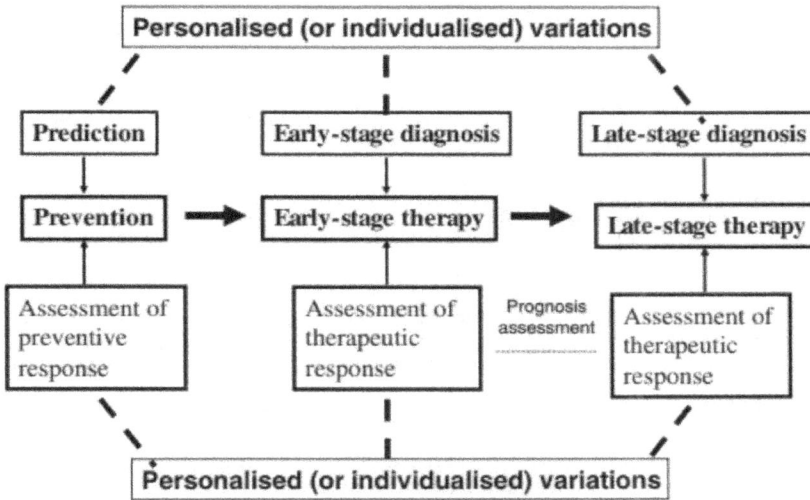

Figure 1.
Variations involved in each aspect of healthcare. Reproduced from Hu et al. [4], with permission from BioMed Central open access article, copyright 2013.

Types	Definition	Application
Type I	This type of biomarker exist a causal relationship with disease, associate with the initiation and development of disease, and can directly address the pathogenesis of disease.	Contribute to the mechanism and therapeutic targets of disease.
Type II	This type of biomarker does not need a causal relationship with the occurrence and development of disease, but requires specificity and a certain amount of change to be easily detected.	Contribute to the prediction, diagnosis, and prognostic assessment.

Table 1.
Concept and categories of biomarkers [9].

to improve the accuracy of cancer diagnosis and therapy [9, 37]. In summary, due to the complex pathophysiological basis of cancer, recognition of molecule-pattern biomarker for precise prediction, diagnosis, and prognostic assessment in cancer is an urgent demand to study and further close to realize precision medicine (PM) and PPPM.

3. Methodology of recognition of multiomics-based pattern biomarkers in cancer

Based on central dogma, genetic changes influence the RNA expression, and cause the alterations of proteins, along with taken into account the changes of metabolite and tumor heterogeneity, all above variations in genome, transcriptome, proteome, metabolome, and radiome are measured with corresponding omics methodology including genomics, transcriptomics, proteomics, metabolomics, and radiomics. Multiomics-generated biomarkers can make up integrative molecule-pattern biomarkers and pattern recognition for cancer treatment. This section mainly addresses the previous mentioned five omics approaches combined with computation biology and systems biology contribute to the development of cancer precise medicine (**Figure 2**) [9].

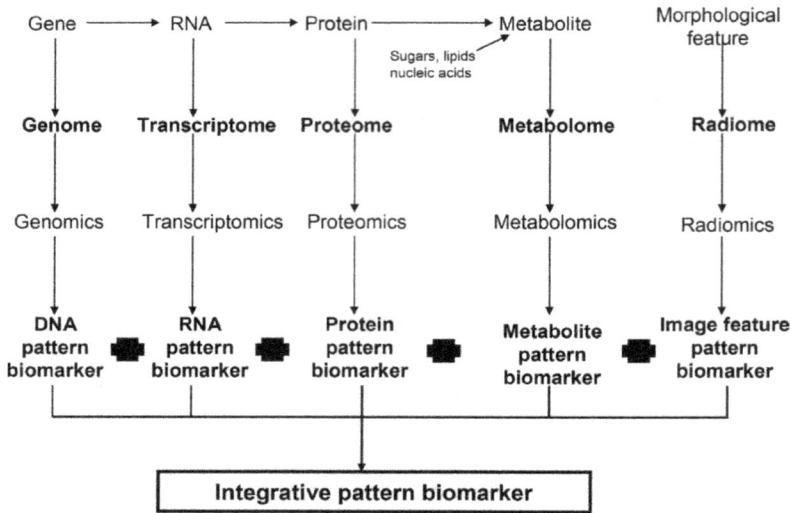

Figure 2.
Different levels of omics-based pattern biomarkers. Modified from Cheng and Zhan [9], with permission from Springer open access article, copyright 2017.

3.1 Genomics

The development of genomics drives the understanding and cognition of cancer. The development of gene sequencing technology is a significant advancement in the field of scientific research. First, based on the method of the previous "plus and minus," Sanger modified and invented the "dideoxy method" for DNA sequencing in 1977 [38–40]. Sanger sequencing acquired many achievements and completed a great work "Human Genome Project." Nevertheless, high cost and low throughput are disadvantages of Sanger sequencing technology [41, 42]. The limit of Sanger sequencing promotes the progression and generation of new sequencing technology. The second-generation sequencing technology has many advantages including higher speed and throughput, higher degree of parallelism, effective utilization of reagents and so on. However, problems still exist, such as the reduction of accuracy of sequencing and relatively higher cost [43, 44]. Due to the presence of shortcomings of the second-generation sequencing technology, the next-generation sequencing (NGS) requires to be discovered. The third-generation of sequencing technology is found to make up for the deficiency of second-generation. For example, PacBio RS and Oxford Nanopore sequencing not only possess fundamental character of the single molecule sequencing, do not need any polymerase chain reaction (PCR) process, availably avoid the PCR bias caused by the system error, and well improve the read length, but also keep the high-throughput and low cost of the second-generation technology [45]. Research demonstrates that accumulation of genomic alternations leads to the occurrence of cancer, which involves small insertions and deletions, base substitutions, copy number alterations (CNA), chromosomal rearrangements, and microbial infections [46]. Besides, a number of polymorphic CNAs have been discovered in the human genome [47]. DNA microarrays, also named as "gene chip" or "DNA chip," obtained a great success that could monitor tens of thousands of one time expression and hundreds of thousands of genes. Single nucleotide polymorphisms (SNPs) are the most common form of DNA variation in the human genome, approximately occurring one time every 100–300 bases [48]. Many studies suggested SNPs might affect the activity of metabolism-related key enzyme, therefore generating effects on tumor progression and drug efficacy. However, with in-depth research, scientists indicated one SNP or a simple CNA could not influence the whole development of the individual process of cancer. The occurrence of a cancer is a result of changes of multiple sites, thus current study is shifting towards several genetic mutation patterns [9]. In addition, breakthrough progress has been made in strategies for obtaining DNA information of tumor tissues. Currently, a novel method found to collect DNA information of tumor tissue is called circulating tumor cell (CTC), which is a general term for all tumor cells in peripheral blood [49]. Compared to tumor tissue samples, blood specimens possess more advantages such as less invasive, easy to acquire, and can be collected repeatedly. It is a typical source of specimens and convenient to operate in clinical practice, so that significantly improves the value of aforementioned method [9]. Circulating tumor DNA (ctDNA) means a tumor cell body that is apoptotic by shedding or released into the circulatory system, and rapid development of gene sequencing results in that it is able to detect in the blood [50]. Therefore, ctDNAs are possible to find key mutation sites and served as biomarkers. Over the past few years, liquid biopsy combined with ctDNA analysis is helpful and beneficial for the molecular diagnosis and monitoring of cancer. Moreover, BEAMing (emulsion, amplification, beads, and magnetics) and CAPP-seq (cancer personalized profiling by deep sequencing) are discovered and used to quantify ctDNA in blood [51, 52]. Furthermore, there are several unknown things about ctDNA including its size, existing form, mechanisms of released into blood stream, and its degradation rate in blood [53]. In summary, the development of genomics provides the method, important information about genome, and impactful biomarkers for diagnosis of cancer and drives the progress of cancer genomics.

3.2 Transcriptomics

Based on the genetic central rule, DNA through self-replication and transcripts to form the mRNAs, and finally translates to be a protein. The mRNA is served as a bridge between gene and protein in biological process and linked genome and phenotype. Once variation of gene sequence of mRNA occurs, the amino acid sequence of the protein will be correspondingly altered. Therefore, the understanding of transcriptomics is important for addressing functional elements of the genome and cognizing the development of cancer. The key goal of transcriptomics is to classify all types of transcripts, reveal the transcriptional structure of the genes, and quantify the expression levels of each transcript during development and under different conditions. Nowadays, many methods are generated to be used for the study of transcriptome, such as hybridization-or sequence-based approaches [54]. In general, the way of nucleic acids with hybridization-based is incubation of fluorescently labeled-complementary DNA (cDNA) from reverse transcription of different mRNAs with a microarray contained genes of interest, then digitized with a dedicated scanner and image analysis and finally gene name, clone identifier, and intensity values are acquired [55]. Furthermore, genomic tiling microarrays are found to provide a more unerring opinion of the transcriptional activities within a genome [56]. Howbeit, there are some disadvantages, like relying on the current knowledge of genome sequence, high background levels owing to cross-hybridization, and both background and saturation of signals resulted in a limited dynamic range of detection [57, 58]. Sequence-based strategy is able to detect cDNA sequence but not depend on the probes. With the development of high-throughput DNA sequencing technique of NGS, a new method used for mapping and quantifying transcriptome is occurred, named RNA-seq. It possesses a lot of advantages, for instance, high throughput, high sensitivity, high resolution, and no reconstructions. RNA-seq is able to analyze the whole transcriptome of any species, including detection of unknown genes or transcripts, exact identification of the cleavage site, and a variable SNP or untranslated region (UTR region) [16]. In another hand, the research field of noncoding RNA (ncRNA) should be paid more attention. The ncRNAs consist of tRNA, rRNA, snoRNA, snRNA, piRNA, miRNA, and lncRNA [59]. Of them, miRNA and lncRNA are familiar and studied more. MicroRNAs, with a sequence of approximately 21 bp, are a kind of small ncRNAs, which take part in multiple cellular functions including proliferation, differentiation, metabolism and apoptosis [60]. In general, TaqMan-based real-time quantitative PCR (RT-qPCR) with separate microRNA-specific primers and probes is used to detect the expression levels of microRNAs. The expression of microRNAs is frequently dysregulated in a cancer-specific manner so that microRNAs are potential to be biomarkers for cancer detection. Many studies demonstrated the microRNAs as biomarkers for prediction, diagnosis, and prognosis for cancer [9]. However, current studies on the function of miRNAs have not yet been fully understood, previous studies of miRNAs have found different types of miRNAs and their effects on oncogenesis and gene expression level of miRNA as antioncogene. In addition, it is predicted that about 30% of protein-encoding genes are regulated by miRNAs [61, 62]. lncRNAs execute multiple functions in cells and are reported as biomarkers in many types of cancers, like breast, lung, gastric, liver, and prostate cancers [63]. The lncRNAs play a vital role in recognition and treatment of cancer. Up to now, the biological effects of lncRNAs are still incompletely clear, but they have already been found to be prolific regulators of many cell processes. Several lncRNAs overlap with gene promoters, thus transcription of these lncRNAs might interfere with nucleosome-deleted regions and histone modifications of nucleosomes in those promoters [64, 65]. Moreover, detection of lncRNA is easily influenced by anticoagulant such as EDTA, and lncRNA is lightly degraded by other substance of the blood so that it cannot be preserved for a long time. More researches are necessary to solve these problems in the future [9].

3.3 Proteomics

Proteins are most direct phenotype characteristics of DNA in biological system. Proteins are related to multiple cellular mechanisms including cell motility, cell growth, cell signaling, and protein metabolic process [66]. The study of proteome is beneficial to the understanding of cancer. The aim of proteomics is to identify proteins and construct protein pathways and networks to characterize information and ultimately understand the functional relevance of proteins in cells or organisms [67]. The proteome is one of the most complex omes among genome, transcriptome, and proteome. The amount of human proteins and their variants or protein species are approximately reached to billions [4]. Furthermore, one gene is corresponded to multiple proteins, known as one gene-multiple proteins model, not one gene-one protein model so that the complexity of proteome is conceivable [68, 69]. So far, only the sequence and copy number of DNAs and RNAs in a genome are able to measure with current technologies. However, a lot of information can be acquired in a proteome, including amino acid sequence, copy number, splicing, variants, post-translational modifications (PTMs), spatial conformation, and spatial redistribution [16]. Proteomics mainly applies to the detection, identification, and quantification of the protein in a defined system (cell, tissue, organ, and organelles). Of detection technologies, gel and gel-free methods are used [68, 69]. Two-dimensional gel electrophoresis (2DGE), two-dimensional difference in gel electrophoresis (2D DIGE), and one-dimensional gel electrophoresis (1DGE) are mainly involved in gel-based methods [69, 70]. When ones want to detect a certain variants of a given protein or a kind of PTM with gel-based methods, a specific antibody is necessary to be used [70–72]. Gel-free methods primarily have hydrophobic interaction chromatography (HIC) to separate large bio-molecules, like proteins, C4 or C5 reverse phase liquid chromatography (RPLC) with 300 Å pore-size particles, capillary electrophoresis (CE)-electrospray ionization-mass spectrometry (CE-ESI-MS), multiplexed gel-eluted liquid fraction entrapment electrophoresis (mGELFrEE; size-based separation) with 8 parallel glass gel column, and weak-cation exchange chromatography (WCX) in combination with HIC in a single column with a single phase (2D-LC; from WCX to HIC mode) [73–80]. Mass spectrometry (MS) plays an important role in identification of protein variants and PTMs, because the amino acid sequence of complete proteins, splicing sites and PTM-sites are able to be determined with MS [69, 71, 81, 82]. Tandem mass spectrometry (MS/MS) can detect amino acid sequence of a protein, and directly authenticate the errors of amino acid sequence, variations, and modifications, which causes character of PTMs and protein variants with different types of mass spectrometers, for instance, matrix-assisted laser desorption ionization-time of flight-time of flight (MALDI-TOF-TOF), LTQ Orbitrap system, triple TOF 5600 or 6600 systems and Fourier transform ion cyclotron resonance (FTICR) with different types of ion fragmentation models including electron capture dissociation (ECD), electron transfer dissociation (ETD) and collision induced dissociation (CID). Different types of samples and research objectives should use identification techniques that are appropriate for them [80]. Quantification of protein is necessary to clarify their biological significance, which is detected with three main methods, including 2DGE-based quantitative methods, label-free quantitative techniques like sequential window acquisition of all theoretical mass spectra (SWATH) and selected/multiple reaction monitoring (SRM/MRM), and stable isotope-labeled quantitative approaches including isobaric tags for relative and absolute quantification iTRAQ [80]. Furthermore, combined with structural proteomics maybe is better for understanding the biological functions in biological systems [83, 84]. Also, the study of the protein-protein interaction analysis and cell signal pathways has become a hot topic. The identification of protein-protein interactions is meaningful for understanding signal transduction mechanisms and establishing intracellular signaling networks [4]. Under pathological conditions, the body can secrete several special proteins owing to the other mRNA synthesis and alternative chromosomal genetic variations involved cancer, diabetes and Alzheimer disease [85]. Therefore, protein is able to be a biomarker and proteomics is an important strategy for the study of cancer.

3.4 Metabolomics

Metabolites and proteins are equally important to understand cancer. Metabolites are small molecules (<1 KDa) produced by metabolism, which can provide functional information that is not directly available from the genome and proteome in cellular and tissue states [86, 87]. Metabolites are derived from lipids, sugars, proteins, and nucleic acids in a given biological system, cell, tissue, or body-fluid [88–90]. The alteration in metabolites is relevant to multiple factors, such as genetic, environment, internal, external, drug, and dietary factors. These metabolic profiles are related to the whole biochemical processes that are the starting, intermediate or final products and provide complex interactions information between the genes and the environment of a given condition [91, 92]. Metabolites may be capable of reflecting physiological and pathological processes and monitoring the progression of a disease, and are helpful to predict, diagnose, and treat [93]. Therefore, metabolomics is a methodology used to study metabolome, refers to identification of biochemical and molecular features of metabolome, among different metabolite interactions between genetic/environmental factors and metabolites, and to assessment of biochemical mechanisms associated with a given conditions like different pathophysiological processes [94]. Generally, two strategies, targeted and untargeted methods, are mainly employed to detect variations in a metabolome [95, 96]. Targeted metabolomics method concentrates on quantification of the variations of the hypothesis-driven known metabolite profiling (like metabolites that are produced from one or more unknown pathways) between or among groups, followed by multivariate statistical analysis and establishment of mathematical model [95, 97]. Up to now, the familiar techniques used for targeted metabolomics are the triple quadrupole mass spectrometry (QqQ-MS) in the SRM/MRM modes with optimized sample extraction and liquid chromatography-mass spectrometry (LC-MS) conditions [98, 99]. The untargeted metabolomics is different from targeted method, which shows in these aspects, such as no hypothesis-driven strategy, and the whole comprehensive study variations of metabolome in a biological system without bias for exploration of metabolite biomarkers for impactful prediction, diagnosis, and prognostic assessment [80, 96]. The current techniques used to qualify and quantify the metabolomic variations are nuclear magnetic resonance (NMR)-based methods and mass spectrometry (MS)-based methods [88, 100–102]. NMR-based methods involve one-dimensional NMR (1D-NMR), two-dimensional NMR (2D-NMR), and three-dimensional NMR (3D-NMR). The way to provide chemical structural and molecular environment information is utilizing the interaction of spin active nuclei (^{13}C, ^{1}H, ^{31}P, ^{19}F) with electromagnetic fields [100, 101]. NMR-based methods possess many advantages, including nondestruction of sample, minimal sample preparation, high reproducibility, relative high throughput, availability of databases, and availability of molecular dynamic and compartmental information with diffusional methods. However, overlapping of metabolites, low sensitivity, and high instrumentation cost are its disadvantages [103]. MS-based methods include direct injection coupled with MS (DIMS), LC-MS, gas chromatography coupled with MS (GC-MS), capillary electrophoresis coupled with MS (CE-MS), and ion mobility coupled with MS (IM-MS) [80]. Aforementioned five MS-based methods have its advantages and limitations, and proper combination helps ones to better study. In clinic, in order to measure variations in a metabolome, the biological samples are extremely complex, including cell, tissue extracts and body-fluid. Serum/plasma and urine are commonly used body-fluid for metabolomics analysis in all diseases because they are very easily acquired and prepared, and almost no injury for patients [88, 104, 105]. Additionally, many researches have reported that cerebrospinal fluid (CSF), saliva, exhaled air, tears, and synovial fluid are likely to be regarded as biomarkers for a specific disease [80]. Metabolites are important source of biomarkers, and metabolomics methods reasonably adopted are beneficial to predict, diagnose, and evaluate for cancer.

3.5 Radiomics

Medical imaging technologies, including computed tomography (CT), positron emission tomography (PET), and magnetic resonance imaging (MRI), are vital to diagnose and check after treatment for cancer. Medical images provide ones with a number of information about tumors, which include location and volume of tumor, probable measurements of diameter, the overall and marginal morphology of the lesion, the relationship with surrounding tissues, internal heterogeneity, CT and PET/CT values, MRI signal height and other values. This information is instructive for the diagnosis of tumors and the decision-making of clinical treatment. However, it is not able to accurately reflect the morphological and behavioral complexities of a tumor, with limitation in the assessment of treatment sensitivity and prognosis [106]. With the rapid development of technology, emerging discipline- radiomics has occurred. Based on excellent computer technology and advanced statistical methods, radiomics achieves high-throughput extraction and conversion of quantitative features of medical data, and make it serve for clinic decision of cancer [16]. Radiomics has enabled medical imaging to achieve a qualitative to quantitative transition and provides guidance for clinical treatment, and a large amount of data has the potential to develop into biomarkers that contribute to further research in cancer.

4. Application of pattern biomarker for PPPM or PM in cancer

Based on the development of multiomics technology, a series of molecular alterations in the levels of genome, transcriptome, proteome, metabolome, and radiome are possible to be detected and measured, which also offer many kinds of potential biomarkers to ones and are beneficial to well understand and study for cancer. In order to improve the treatment effect and approach PPPM or PM in cancer, the methodology of recognition of multiomics-based molecule-pattern biomarker is presented. The concept "pattern biomarker" refers to several biomarkers make up a pattern for precise prediction, diagnosis, and prognostic assessment in cancer, which can be derived from genome, transcriptome, proteome, metabolome, or radiome, and each pattern biomarker is able to be used as a biomarker for recognition, therapy, and other-related research of cancer. Many researches prove that the use of more biomarkers can increase the accuracy of understanding for cancer. For instance, based on somatic cell gene copy number aberrations, the alterations of gene expression analyzed with genomic and transcriptomic data and long-term clinical outcomes indicated several potentially important targeted therapeutic response-related events and mentioned a novel molecular classification of breast cancer patients [107]. Genomic combined with proteomic data analysis revealed that PI3K pathway aberrations are popular in hormone receptor-positive breast cancer, which provides new idea for clinically targeted therapy [108]. Tissue transcriptomics and urine metabolomics integrated analysis identified four urinary biomarkers that are more reliable compared to biomarkers derived from single omics

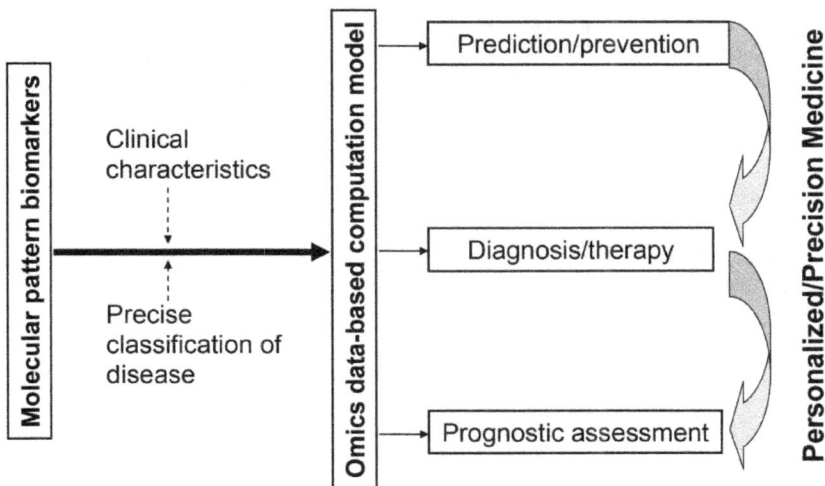

Figure 3.
Application of pattern biomarker in personalized medicine or precision medicine.

[109]. Comprehensive analysis of transcriptomic and proteomic data suggested a highly significant enrichment of gonadotropin-releasing hormone (GnRH) signaling pathway that was not deciphered with single omics dataset in glioblastomas, which proved the necessity of multiomics research [110]. In addition, the failure of sorafenib-treated HCCs was employed with an integrated quantitative proteomics and phosphoproteomics analysis, and found that the targeted drug can effectively inhibit its target kinase in Raf-Erk-Rsk pathway, but the downstream targets of Rsk-2 (eIF4B, filamin-A, and so on) were not affected, suggesting that they may be replaced by another active pathway and lead to treatment failure [111]. However, there are also many challenges needed to be faced. Considering the tumor heterogeneity, individual difference, different stages of tumor development, the recurrence of tumor, and so on, one designs an ideal model for prediction, prognosis, and prognostic assessment of cancer in order to further realize PPPM or PM (**Figure 3**).

5. Conclusion

Cancer is a complex whole-body chronic disease, is involved in multiple causes, multiple processes, and multiple consequences. On the contrary, the complexity of cancer exactly provides ones with more opportunities for PPPM or PM in cancer. The rapid development of genomics, transcriptomics, proteomics, metabolomics, and radiomics in combination with advanced computation biology and systems biology drives the development of pattern recognition to find reliable and effective molecular pattern biomarkers for cancer treatment, and further achieves PPPM or PM. Multiomics integration analysis is beneficial to better understand cell malignant transformation and tumor progression, clarify molecular mechanisms of a cancer, discover novel biomarkers and targeted drugs, and improve the effect of targeted therapies.

Acknowledgements

The authors acknowledge the financial supports from the Xiangya Hospital Funds for Talent Introduction (to X.Z.), the Hunan Provincial "Hundred Talent Plan" program (to X.Z.), the National Natural Science Foundation of China (Grant No. 81572278 and 81272798 to X.Z.), China "863" Plan Project (Grant No. 2014AA020610-1 to X.Z.), and the Hunan Provincial Natural Science Foundation of China (Grant No. 14JJ7008 to X.Z.).

Conflict of interest

We declare that we have no financial and personal relationships with other people or organizations.

Author's contributions

Z.T. analyzed references and wrote manuscript draft of the book chapter. C.T. M.L. participated in collection of references and analysis of data. X.Z. conceived the concept, designed the book chapter, and critically revised/wrote the book chapter, coordinated and was responsible for the correspondence work and financial support.

Acronyms and abbreviations

CAPP-seq	cancer personalized profiling by deep sequencing
cDNA	complementary DNA
CE	capillary electrophoresis
CE-MS	capillary electrophoresis coupled with MS
CE-ESI-MS	capillary electrophoresis-electrospray ionization-massspectrometry
CID	collision induced dissociation
CNA	copy number alterations
CSF	cerebrospinal fluid
CT	computed tomography
CTC	circulating tumor cell
ctDNA	circulating tumor DNA
DIMS	direct injection coupled with MS
ECM	extracellular matrix
ECD	electron capture dissociation
ETD	electron transfer dissociation
FTICR	Fourier transform ion cyclotron resonance
GC-MS	gas chromatography coupled with MS
GnRH	gonadotropin-releasing hormone
HIC	hydrophobic interaction chromatography
lncRNAs	long noncoding RNAs
IM-MS	ion mobility coupled with MS
iTRAQ	isobaric tags for relative and absolute quantification
LC-MS	liquid chromatography-mass spectrometry
MAPK	mitogen-activated protein kinase
mGELFrEE	multiplexed gel-eluted liquid fraction entrapment electrophoresis
mRNA	messenger RNA
MS	mass spectrometry
MALDI-TOF-TOF	matrix-assisted laser desorption ionization-time of flight-time of flight
MRI	magnetic resonance imaging
mTOR	mammalian target of rapamycin
ncRNA	noncoding RNA
NGS	next-generation sequencing
NMR	nuclear magnetic resonance
NPC	nasopharyngeal carcinoma
1DGE	one-dimensional gel electrophoresis
PCR	polymerase chain reaction
PET	positron emission tomography
PM	precision medicine
PPPM	predictive, preventive, and personalized medicine
PI3K/Akt	phosphoinositide 3-kinase/protein kinase B
PTMs	post-translational modifications
QqQ-MS	quadrupole mass spectrometry
RPLC	reverse phase liquid chromatography
RT-qPCR	real-time quantitative PCR
SNPs	single nucleotide polymorphisms
STAT3	signal transducer, and activator of transcription 3
SWATH	sequential window acquisition of all theoretical mass spectra

SRM/MRM	selected/multiple reaction monitoring
1D-NMR	one-dimensional NMR
2D-NMR	two-dimensional NMR
3D-NMR	three-dimensional NMR
2DGE	two-dimensional gel electrophoresis
2D DIGE	two-dimensional difference in gel electrophoresis
MS/MS	Tandem mass spectrometry
UTR region	untranslated region
WCX	weak-cation exchange chromatography

Author details

Xanquan Zhan*, Tian Zhou, Tingting Cheng and Miaolong Lu
Key Laboratory of Cancer Proteomics of Chinese Ministry of Health, Xiangya
Hospital, Central South University, Changsha, China

*Address all correspondence to: yjzhan2011@gmail.com

IntechOpen

References

[1] Block KI, Gyllenhaal C, Lowe L, Amedei A, ARMR A, Amin A, et al. A broad-spectrum integrative design for cancer prevention and therapy. Seminars in Cancer Biology. 2015;**35**(Suppl):S276-S304. DOI: 10.1016/j.semcancer.2015.09.007

[2] Friedl P, Alexander S. Cancer invasion and the microenvironment: Plasticity and reciprocity. Cell. 2011;**147**:992-1009. DOI: 10.1016/j.cell.2011.11.016

[3] Maximo V, Lima J, Prazeres H, Soares P, Sobrinho-Simoes M. The biology and the genetics of Hurthle cell tumors of the thyroid. Endocrine-Related Cancer. 2012;**19**:R131-R147. DOI: 10.1530/ERC-11-0354

[4] Hu R, Wang X, Zhan X. Multi-parameter systematic strategies for predictive, preventive and personalised medicine in cancer. The EPMA Journal. 2013;**4**:2. DOI: 10.1186/1878-5085-4-2

[5] Kang M, Buckley YM, Lowe AJ. Testing the role of genetic factors across multiple independent invasions of the shrub scotch broom (*Cytisus scoparius*). Molecular Ecology. 2007;**16**:4662-4673

[6] Jobling MA. The impact of recent events on human genetic diversity. Philosophical Transactions of the Royal Society of London. Series B, Biological Sciences. 2012;**367**:793-799. DOI: 10.1098/rstb.2011.0297

[7] Vogelstein B, Papadopoulos N, Velculescu VE, Zhou S, Diaz LA Jr, Kinzler KW. Cancer genome landscapes. Science. 2013;**339**:1546-1558. DOI: 10.1126/science.1235122

[8] Hoth M. CRAC channels, calcium, and cancer in light of the driver and passenger concept. Biochimica et Biophysica Acta. 2016;**1863**:1408-1417. DOI: 10.1016/j.bbamcr.2015.12.009

[9] Cheng T, Zhan X. Pattern recognition for predictive, preventive, and personalized medicine in cancer. The EPMA Journal. 2017;**8**:51-60. DOI: 10.1007/s13167-017-0083-9

[10] Wagner PD, Srivastava S. New paradigms in translational science research in cancer biomarkers. Translational Research. 2012;**159**: 343-353. DOI: 10.1016/j.trsl.2012.01.015

[11] Canonica GW, Bachert C, Hellings P, Ryan D, Valovirta E, Wickman M, et al. Allergen immunotherapy (AIT): A prototype of precision medicine. World Allergy Organization Journal. 2015;**8**:31. DOI: 10.1186/s40413-015-0079-7

[12] Biomarkers Definitions Working Group. Biomarkers and surrogate endpoints: Preferred definitions and conceptual framework. Clinical Pharmacology and Therapeutics. 2001;**69**:89-95. DOI: 10.1067/mcp.2001.113989

[13] Zhai XH, Yu JK, Yang FQ, Zheng S. Identification of a new protein biomarker for colorectal cancer diagnosis. Molecular Medicine Reports. 2012;**6**:444-448. DOI: 10.3892/mmr.2012.923

[14] Taylor DR, Pavord ID. Biomarkers in the assessment and management of airways diseases. Postgraduate Medical Journal. 2008;**84**:628-634; quiz 633. DOI: 10.1136/pgmj.2008.069864

[15] Manolio TA. Genomewide association studies and assessment of the risk of disease. The New England Journal of Medicine. 2010;**363**:166-176. DOI: 10.1056/NEJMra0905980

[16] Lu M, Zhan X. The crucial role of multiomic approach in cancer research and clinically relevant outcomes. The EPMA Journal. 2018;**9**:77-102. DOI: doi.org/10.1007/s13167-018-0128-8

[17] Gonzalez-Angulo AM, Iwamoto T, Liu S, Chen H, Do KA, Hortobagyi GN, et al. Gene expression, molecular class changes, and pathway analysis after neoadjuvant systemic therapy for breast cancer. Clinical Cancer Research. 2012;**18**:1109-1119. DOI: 10.1158/1078-0432.CCR-11-2762

[18] Nosho K, Baba Y, Tanaka N, Shima K, Hayashi M, Meyerhardt JA, et al. Tumour-infiltrating T-cell subsets, molecular changes in colorectal cancer, and prognosis: Cohort study and literature review. The Journal of Pathology. 2010;**222**:350-366. DOI: 10.1002/path.2774

[19] Sheltzer JM, Torres EM, Dunham MJ, Amon A. Transcriptional consequences of aneuploidy. Proceedings of the National Academy of Sciences of the United States of America. 2012;**109**:12644-12649. DOI: 10.1073/pnas.1209227109

[20] Gould CM, Courtneidge SA. Regulation of invadopodia by the tumor microenvironment. Cell Adhesion & Migration. 2014;**8**:226-235

[21] Hanahan D, Weinberg RA. Hallmarks of cancer: The next generation. Cell. 2011;**144**:646-674. DOI: 10.1016/j.cell.2011.02.013

[22] Zhan X, Desiderio DM. The use of variations in proteomes to predict, prevent, and personalize treatment for clinically nonfunctional pituitary adenomas. The EPMA Journal. 2010;**1**:439-459. DOI: 10.1007/s13167-010-0028-z

[23] Longo DL. Tumor heterogeneity and personalized medicine. The New England Journal of Medicine. 2012;**366**:956-957. DOI: 10.1056/NEJMe1200656

[24] Moreno CS, Evans CO, Zhan X, Okor M, Desiderio DM, Oyesiku NM. Novel molecular signaling and classification of human clinically nonfunctional pituitary adenomas identified by gene expression profiling and proteomic analyses. Cancer Research. 2005;**65**:10214-10222

[25] Samuel N, Hudson TJ. Translating genomics to the clinic: Implications of cancer heterogeneity. Clinical Chemistry. 2013;**59**:127-137. DOI: 10.1373/clinchem.2012.184580

[26] Almendro V, Marusyk A, Polyak K. Cellular heterogeneity and molecular evolution in cancer. Annual Review of Pathology. 2013;**8**:277-302. DOI: 10.1146/annurev-pathol-020712-163923

[27] Julien S, Merino-Trigo A, Lacroix L, Pocard M, Goéré D, Mariani P, et al. Characterization of a large panel of patient-derived tumor xenografts representing the clinical heterogeneity of human colorectal cancer. Clinical Cancer Research. 2012;**18**:5314-5328. DOI: 10.1158/1078-0432.CCR-12-0372

[28] Damia G, D'Incalci M. Genetic instability influences drug response in cancer cells. Current Drug Targets. 2010;**11**:1317-1324

[29] Marusyk A, Almendro V, Polyak K. Intra-tumour heterogeneity: A looking glass for cancer? Nature Reviews. Cancer. 2012;**12**:323-334. DOI: 10.1038/nrc3261

[30] George O, Koob GF. Individual differences in prefrontal cortex function and the transition from drug use to drug dependence. Neuroscience and Biobehavioral Reviews. 2010;**35**:232-247. DOI: 10.1016/j.neubiorev.2010.05.002

[31] Zhan X, Desiderio DM. Signaling pathway networks mined from human pituitary adenoma proteomics data. BMC Medical Genomics. 2010;**3**:13. DOI: 10.1186/1755-8794-3-13

[32] Laplante M, Sabatini DM. mTOR signaling in growth control and disease.

Cell. 2012;**149**:274-293. DOI: 10.1016/j.
cell.2012.03.017

[33] Chen J. Multiple signal pathways
in obesity-associated cancer. Obesity
Reviews. 2011;**12**:1063-1070. DOI:
10.1111/j.1467-789X.2011.00917.x

[34] Janku F, Wheler JJ, Westin SN,
Moulder SL, Naing A, Tsimberidou AM,
et al. PI3K/AKT/mTOR inhibitors in
patients with breast and gynecologic
malignancies harboring PIK3CA
mutations. Journal of Clinical Oncology.
2012;**30**:777-782. DOI: 10.1200/
JCO.2011.36.1196

[35] Palumbo MO, Kavan P, Miller WH
Jr, Panasci L, Assouline S, Johnson N,
et al. Systemic cancer therapy:
Achievements and challenges that lie
ahead. Frontiers in Pharmacology.
2013;**4**:57. DOI: 10.3389/fphar.2013.
00057

[36] Liu FF. Novel gene therapy
approach for nasopharyngeal
carcinoma. Seminars in Cancer Biology.
2002;**12**:505-515

[37] Cheon S. Probability concepts
and distributions for analyzing large
biological data. In: Lee JK, editor.
Statistical Bioinformatics for Biomedical
and Life Science Researchers. Hoboken:
Willey; 2010. pp. 7-56

[38] Sanger F, Nicklen S, Coulson
AR. DNA sequencing with chain-
terminating inhibitors. Proceedings
of the National Academy of Sciences
of the United States of America.
1977;**74**:5463-5467

[39] Sanger F, Coulson AR. A rapid
method for determining sequences in
DNA by primed synthesis with DNA
polymerase. Journal of Molecular
Biology. 1975;**94**:441-448

[40] Sanger F. Determination
of nucleotide sequences in
DNA. Bioscience Reports. 1981;**1**:3-18

[41] Tran B, Dancey JE, Kamel-Reid S,
McPherson JD, Bedard PL, Brown AM,
et al. Cancer genomics: Technology,
discovery, and translation. Journal of
Clinical Oncology. 2012;**30**:647-660.
DOI: 10.1200/JCO.2011.39.2316

[42] Metzker ML. Sequencing
technologies—The next generation.
Nature Reviews. Genetics. 2010;**11**:
31-46. DOI: 10.1038/nrg2626

[43] Shendure J, Ji H. Next-generation
DNA sequencing. Nature Biotechnology.
2008;**26**:1135-1145. DOI: 10.1038/
nbt1486

[44] Ansorge WJ. Next-generation
DNA sequencing techniques. New
Biotechnology. 2009;**25**:195-203. DOI:
10.1016/j.nbt.2008.12.009

[45] Niedringhaus TP, Milanova D, Kerby
MB, Snyder MP, Barron AE. Landscape
of next-generation sequencing
technologies. Analytical Chemistry.
2011;**83**:4327-4341. DOI: 10.1021/
ac2010857

[46] Meyerson M, Gabriel S, Getz G.
Advances in understanding cancer
genomes through second-generation
sequencing. Nature Reviews. Genetics.
2010;**11**:685-696. DOI: 10.1038/nrg2841

[47] Pique-Regi R, Monso-Varona
J, Ortega A, Seeger RC, Triche TJ,
Asgharzadeh S. Sparse representation
and Bayesian detection of genome copy
number alterations from microarray
data. Bioinformatics. 2008;**24**:309-318.
DOI: 10.1093/bioinformatics/btm601

[48] Sherry ST, Ward MH, Kholodov M,
Baker J, Phan L, Smigielski EM, et al.
dbSNP: The NCBI database of genetic
variation. Nucleic Acids Research.
2001;**29**:308-311

[49] Sorenson GD, Pribish DM, Valone
FH, Memoli VA, Bzik DJ, Yao SL.
Soluble normal and mutated DNA
sequences from single-copy genes in

human blood. Cancer Epidemiology, Biomarkers & Prevention. 1994;**3**:67-71

[50] Bettegowda C, Sausen M, Leary RJ, Kinde I, Wang Y, Agrawal N, et al. Detection of circulating tumor DNA in early- and late-stage human malignancies. Science Translational Medicine. 2014;**6**:224ra24. DOI: 10.1126/scitranslmed.3007094

[51] Diehl F, Schmidt K, Choti MA, Romans K, Goodman S, Li M, et al. Circulating mutant DNA to assess tumor dynamics. Nature Medicine. 2008;**14**:985-990. DOI: 10.1038/nm.1789

[52] Newman AM, Bratman SV, To J, Wynne JF, Eclov NC, Modlin LA, et al. An ultrasensitive method for quantitating circulating tumor DNA with broad patient coverage. Nature Medicine. 2014;**20**:548-554. DOI: 10.1038/nm.3519

[53] Cheng F, Su L, Qian C. Circulating tumor DNA: A promising biomarker in the liquid biopsy of cancer. Oncotarget. 2016;**7**:48832-48841. DOI: 10.18632/oncotarget.9453

[54] Wang Z, Gerstein M, Snyder M. RNA-Seq: A revolutionary tool for transcriptomics. Nature Reviews. Genetics. 2009;**10**:57-63. DOI: 10.1038/nrg2484

[55] Duggan DJ, Bittner M, Chen Y, Meltzer P, Trent JM. Expression profiling using cDNA microarrays. Nature Genetics. 1999;**21**(1 Suppl):10-14

[56] Yazaki J, Gregory BD, Ecker JR. Mapping the genome landscape using tiling array technology. Current Opinion in Plant Biology. 2007;**10**:534-542

[57] Mishra PJ. MicroRNA polymorphisms: A giant leap towards personalized medicine. Personalized Medicine. 2009;**6**:119-125

[58] Wu X, Weng L, Li X, Guo C, Pal SK, Jin JM, et al. Identification of a 4-microRNA signature for clear cell renal cell carcinoma metastasis and prognosis. PLoS One. 2012;**7**:e35661. DOI: 10.1371/journal.pone.0035661

[59] Alahari SV, Eastlack SC, Alahari SK. Role of long noncoding RNAs in neoplasia: Special emphasis on prostate cancer. International Review of Cell and Molecular Biology. 2016;**324**:229-254. DOI: 10.1016/bs.ircmb.2016.01.004

[60] Reid JF, Sokolova V, Zoni E, Lampis A, Pizzamiglio S, Bertan C, et al. miRNA profiling in colorectal cancer highlights miR-1 involvement in MET-dependent proliferation. Molecular Cancer Research. 2012;**10**:504-515. DOI: 10.1158/1541-7786

[61] Li Y, Cao H, Jiao Z, Pakala SB, Sirigiri DN, Li W, et al. Carcinoembryonic antigen interacts with TGF-{beta} receptor and inhibits TGF-{beta} signaling in colorectal cancers. Cancer Research. 2010;**70**:8159-8168. DOI: 10.1158/0008-5472

[62] Liu M, Li CF, Chen HS, Lin LQ, Zhang CP, Zhao JL, et al. Differential expression of proteomics models of colorectal cancer, colorectal benign disease and healthy controls. Proteome Science. 2010;**8**:16. DOI: 10.1186/1477-5956-8-16

[63] Houseley J, Rubbi L, Grunstein M, Tollervey D, Vogelauer M. A ncRNA modulates histone modification and mRNA induction in the yeast GAL gene cluster. Molecular Cell. 2008;**32**:685-695. DOI: 10.1016/j.molcel.2008.09.027

[64] Pauli A, Valen E, Lin MF, Garber M, Vastenhouw NL, Levin JZ, et al. Systematic identification of long noncoding RNAs expressed during zebrafish embryogenesis. Genome Research. 2012;**22**:577-591. DOI: 10.1101/gr.133009.111

[65] Ponting CP, Oliver PL, Reik W. Evolution and functions of long

noncoding RNAs. Cell. 2009;**136**: 629-641. DOI: 10.1016/j.cell.2009.02.006

[66] Karley D, Gupta D, Tiwari A. Biomarker for cancer: A great promise for future. World Journal of Oncology. 2011;**2**:151-157. DOI: 10.4021/wjon352w

[67] Horgan RP, Kenny LC. 'Omic' technologies: Genomics, transcriptomics, proteomics and metabolomics. The Obstetrician and Gynaecologist. 2011;**13**:189-195

[68] Stastna M, Van Eyk JE. Analysis of protein isoforms: Can we do it better? Proteomics. 2012;**12**:2937-2948. DOI: 10.1002/pmic.201200161

[69] Zhan X, Giorgianni F, Desiderio DM. Proteomics analysis of growth hormone isoforms in the human pituitary. Proteomics. 2005;**5**:1228-1241

[70] Kohler M, Thomas A, Püschel K, Schänzer W, Thevis M. Identification of human pituitary growth hormone variants by mass spectrometry. Journal of Proteome Research. 2009;**8**: 1071-1076. DOI: 10.1021/pr800945b

[71] Peng F, Li J, Guo T, Yang H, Li M, Sang S, et al. Nitroproteins in human astrocytomas discovered by gel electrophoresis and tandem mass spectrometry. Journal of the American Society for Mass Spectrometry. 2015;**26**:2062-2076. DOI: 10.1007/ s13361-015-1270-3

[72] Ono M, Matsubara J, Honda K, Sakuma T, Hashiguchi T, Nose H, et al. Prolyl 4-hydroxylation of alpha-fibrinogen: A novel protein modification revealed by plasma proteomics. The Journal of Biological Chemistry. 2009;**284**:29041-29049. DOI: 10.1074/jbc.M109.041749

[73] Goheen SC, Engelhorn SC. Hydrophobic interaction high-performance liquid chromatography of proteins. Journal of Chromatography. 1984;**317**:55-65

[74] Cummins PM, O'Connor BF. Hydrophobic interaction chromatography. Methods in Molecular Biology. 2011;**681**:431-437. DOI: 10.1007/978-1-60761-913-0_24

[75] Hong G, Gao M, Yan G, Guan X, Tao Q, Zhang X. Optimization of two-dimensional high performance liquid chromatographic columns for highly efficient separation of intact proteins. Se Pu. 2010;**28**:158-162

[76] Staub A, Zurlino D, Rudaz S, Veuthey JL, Guillarme D. Analysis of peptides and proteins using sub-2 μm fully porous and sub 3-μm shell particles. Journal of Chromatography. A. 2011;**1218**:8903-8914. DOI: 10.1016/j. chroma.2011.07.051

[77] Tran JC, Doucette AA. Multiplexed size separation of intact proteins in solution phase for mass spectrometry. Analytical Chemistry. 2009;**81**: 6201-6209. DOI: 10.1021/ac900729r

[78] Sikanen T, Aura S, Franssila S, Kotiaho T, Kostiainen R. Microchip capillary electrophoresis-electrospray ionization-mass spectrometry of intact proteins using uncoated Ormocomp microchips. Analytica Chimica Acta. 2012;**711**:69-76. DOI: 10.1016/j. aca.2011.10.059

[79] Geng X, Ke C, Chen G, Liu P, Wang F, Zhang H, et al. On-line separation of native proteins by two-dimensional liquid chromatography using a single column. Journal of Chromatography. A. 2009;**1216**:3553-3562. DOI: 10.1016/j. chroma.2009.01.085

[80] Zhan X, Long Y, Lu M. Exploration of variations in proteome and metabolome for predictive diagnostics and personalized treatment algorithms: Innovative approach and examples for potential clinical application. Journal of Proteomics. 2018;**188**:30-40. DOI: 10.1016/j. jprot.2017.08.020

[81] Guo T, Wang X, Li M, Yang H, Li L, Peng F, et al. Identification of glioblastoma phosphotyrosine-containing proteins with two-dimensional western blotting and tandem mass spectrometry. BioMed Research International. 2015;**2015**:134050. DOI: 10.1155/2015/134050

[82] Zhan X, Desiderio DM. The human pituitary nitroproteome: Detection of nitrotyrosyl-proteins with two-dimensional western blotting, and amino acid sequence determination with mass spectrometry. Biochemical and Biophysical Research Communications. 2004;**325**:1180-1186

[83] Zhan X, Wang X, Desiderio DM. Mass spectrometry analysis of nitrotyrosine-containing proteins. Mass Spectrometry Reviews. 2015;**34**: 423-448. DOI: 10.1002/mas.21413

[84] Hyung SJ, Ruotolo BT. Integrating mass spectrometry of intact protein complexes into structural proteomics. Proteomics. 2012;**12**:1547-1564. DOI: 10.1002/pmic.201100520

[85] Deschoolmeester V, Baay M, Specenier P, Lardon F, Vermorken JB. A review of the most promising biomarkers in colorectal cancer: One step closer to targeted therapy. The Oncologist. 2010;**15**:699-731. DOI: 10.1634/theoncologist.2010-0025

[86] Holmes E, Wilson ID, Nicholson JK. Metabolic phenotyping in health and disease. Cell. 2008;**134**:714-717. DOI: 10.1016/j.cell.2008.08.026

[87] Patti GJ, Yanes O, Siuzdak G. Innovation: Metabolomics: The apogee of the omics trilogy. Nature Reviews. Molecular Cell Biology. 2012;**13**:263-269. DOI: 10.1038/nrm3314

[88] Khamis MM, Adamko DJ, El-Aneed A. Mass spectrometric based approaches in urine metabolomics and biomarker

discovery. Mass Spectrometry Reviews. 2017;**36**:115-134. DOI: 10.1002/mas.21455

[89] Dunn WB, Broadhurst DI, Atherton HJ, Goodacre R, Griffin JL. Systems level studies of mammalian metabolomes: The roles of mass spectrometry and nuclear magnetic resonance spectroscopy. Chemical Society Reviews. 2011;**40**:387-426. DOI: 10.1039/b906712b

[90] Nicholson JK, Lindon JC, Holmes E. 'Metabonomics': Understanding the metabolic responses of living systems to pathophysiological stimuli via multivariate statistical analysis of biological NMR spectroscopic data. Xenobiotica. 1999;**29**:1181-1189

[91] Nicholson JK. Global systems biology, personalized medicine and molecular epidemiology. Molecular Systems Biology. 2006;**2**:52

[92] Mirsaeidi M, Banoei MM, Winston BW, Schraufnagel DE. Metabolomics: Applications and promise in mycobacterial disease. Annals of the American Thoracic Society. 2015;**12**:1278-1287. DOI: 10.1513/AnnalsATS.201505-279PS

[93] Everett JR. Pharmacometabonomics in humans: A new tool for personalized medicine. Pharmacogenomics. 2015;**16**:737-754. DOI: 10.2217/pgs.15.20

[94] Tebani A, Abily-Donval L, Afonso C, Marret S, Bekri S. Clinical metabolomics: The new metabolic window for inborn errors of metabolism investigations in the post-genomic era. International Journal of Molecular Sciences. 2016;**17**. DOI: 10.3390/ijms17071167

[95] Siskos AP, Jain P, Römisch-Margl W, Bennett M, Achaintre D, Asad Y, et al. Interlaboratory reproducibility of a targeted metabolomics platform for analysis of human serum and plasma.

Analytical Chemistry. 2017;**89**:656-665. DOI: 10.1021/acs.analchem.6b02930

[96] Mizuno H, Ueda K, Kobayashi Y, Tsuyama N, Todoroki K, Min JZ, et al. The great importance of normalization of LC-MS data for highly-accurate non-targeted metabolomics. Biomedical Chromatography. 2017;**31**:e3864. DOI: 10.1002/bmc.3864

[97] Kitteringham NR, Jenkins RE, Lane CS, Elliott VL, Park BK. Multiple reaction monitoring for quantitative biomarker analysis in proteomics and metabolomics. Journal of Chromatography. B, Analytical Technologies in the Biomedical and Life Sciences. 2009;**877**:1229-1239. DOI: 10.1016/j.jchromb.2008.11.013

[98] Zhou J, Yin Y. Strategies for large-scale targeted metabolomics quantification by liquid chromatography-mass spectrometry. The Analyst. 2016;**141**:6362-6373

[99] Guo B, Chen B, Liu A, Zhu W, Yao S. Liquid chromatography-mass spectrometric multiple reaction monitoring-based strategies for expanding targeted profiling towards quantitative metabolomics. Current Drug Metabolism. 2012;**13**:1226-1243

[100] Kruk J, Doskocz M, Jodłowska E, Zacharzewska A, Łakomiec J, Czaja K, et al. NMR techniques in metabolomic studies: A quick overview on examples of utilization. Applied Magnetic Resonance. 2017;**48**:1-21. DOI: 10.1007/s00723-016-0846-9

[101] Marchand J, Martineau E, Guitton Y, Dervilly-Pinel G, Giraudeau P. Multidimensional NMR approaches towards highly resolved, sensitive and high-throughput quantitative metabolomics. Current Opinion in Biotechnology. 2017;**43**:49-55. DOI: 10.1016/j.copbio.2016.08.004

[102] Naz S, Moreira dos Santos DC, García A, Barbas C. Analytical protocols based on LC-MS, GC-MS and CE-MS for nontargeted metabolomics of biological tissues. Bioanalysis. 2014;**6**:1657-1677. DOI: 10.4155/bio.14.119

[103] Markley JL, Brüschweiler R, Edison AS, Eghbalnia HR, Powers R, Raftery D, et al. The future of NMR-based metabolomics. Current Opinion in Biotechnology. 2017;**43**:34-40. DOI: 10.1016/j.copbio.2016.08.001

[104] Dunn WB, Broadhurst D, Begley P, Zelena E, Francis-McIntyre S, Anderson N, et al. Procedures for large-scale metabolic profiling of serum and plasma using gas chromatography and liquid chromatography coupled to mass spectrometry. Nature Protocols. 2011;**6**:1060-1083. DOI: 10.1038/nprot.2011.335

[105] Want EJ, Wilson ID, Gika H, Theodoridis G, Plumb RS, Shockcor J, et al. Global metabolic profiling procedures for urine using UPLC-MS. Nature Protocols. 2010;**5**:1005-1018. DOI: 10.1038/nprot.2010.50

[106] Kumar V, Gu Y, Basu S, Berglund A, Eschrich SA, Schabath MB, et al. Radiomics: The process and the challenges. Magnetic Resonance Imaging. 2012;**30**:1234-1248. DOI: 10.1016/j.mri.2012.06.010

[107] Curtis C, Shah SP, Chin SF, Turashvili G, Rueda OM, Dunning MJ, et al. The genomic and transcriptomic architecture of 2,000 breast tumours reveals novel subgroups. Nature. 2012;**486**:346-352. DOI: 10.1038/nature10983

[108] Stemke-Hale K, Gonzalez-Angulo AM, Lluch A, Neve RM, Kuo WL, Davies M, et al. An integrative genomic and proteomic analysis of PIK3CA, PTEN, and AKT mutations in breast cancer. Cancer Research. 2008;**68**:6084-6091. DOI: 10.1158/0008-5472.CAN-07-6854

[109] Nam H, Chung BC, Kim Y, Lee K, Lee D. Combining tissue transcriptomics and urine metabolomics for breast cancer biomarker identification. Bioinformatics. 2009;**25**:3151-3157. DOI: 10.1093/bioinformatics/btp558

[110] Jayaram S, Gupta MK, Raju R, Gautam P, Sirdeshmukh R. Multi-omics data integration and mapping of altered kinases to pathways reveal gonadotropin hormone signaling in glioblastoma. OMICS International. 2016;**20**:736-746

[111] Dazert E, Colombi M, Boldanova T, Moes S, Adametz D, Quagliata L, et al. Quantitative proteomics and phosphoproteomics on serial tumor biopsies from a sorafenib-treated HCC patient. Proceedings of the National Academy of Sciences of the United States of America. 2016;**113**:1381-1386. DOI: 10.1073/pnas.1523434113

Chapter 5

HCV Genotyping with Concurrent Profiling of Resistance-Associated Variants by NGS Analysis

Kok-Siong Poon, Julian Wei-Tze Tang
and Evelyn Siew-Chuan Koay

Abstract

Determination of viral characteristics including genotype (GT), subtype (ST) and resistance-associated variants (RAVs) profile is important in assigning direct-acting antivirals regimes in HCV patients. To help achieve the best clinical management of HCV patients, a routine diagnostic laboratory should aim at reporting accurate viral GT/ST and RAVs using a reliable diagnostic platform of choice. A laboratory study was conducted to evaluate performance characteristics of a new commercial next-generation sequencing (NGS)-based HCV genotyping assay in comparison to another widely used commercial line probe assay for HCV genotyping. Information on RAVs from deeply sequenced NS3, NS5A and NS5B regions in samples classified as HCV 1a and 1b was harnessed from the fully automated software. Perfect (100%) concordance at HCV genotype level was achieved in GT2 (N = 13), GT3 (N = 55) and GT5 (N = 7). NGS refined the ST assignment in GTs 1, 4 and 6, and resolved previously indeterminate GTs reported by line probe assay. NGS was found to have consistent intra- and inter-run reproducibility in terms of genotyping, subtyping and RAVs identification. Detection of infections with multiple HCV GTs or STs is feasible by NGS. Deep sequencing allows sensitive identification of RAVs in the GT 1a and 1b NS3, NS5A and NS5B regions, but the list of target RAVs is not exhaustive.

Keywords: resistance-associated variants, next-generation sequencing, hepatitis C, HCV genotyping, NGS

1. Introduction

Due to the genetic diversity of the hepatitis C virus (HCV), its accurate genotyping is still currently challenging despite the use of modern molecular techniques. In addition to the six widely-recognised HCV genotypes, a newly identified genotype (GT) 7 was reported in 2015 [1]. Molecular methods including reverse hybridization, real-time PCR and Sanger sequencing are commonly utilised for HCV genotyping and subtyping in clinical laboratories. HCV genotype and subtype (ST) have been the critical factors in decision-making for administering interferon-based therapies for the past decade [2]. According to the latest AASLD guidelines [3], determination of viral characteristics including GT, ST and resistance-associated variants (RAVs) profile is important in assigning direct-acting antivirals (DAAs) regimes in HCV patients.

To help achieve the best clinical management of HCV patients, a routine diagnostic laboratory should aim at minimising reporting out non-informative HCV genotyping results which are due to inherent limitations of the diagnostic platform of choice. In general, about 2–8.5% of HCV positive samples have been reported to carry "indeterminate" GTs by several commercial assays [4–9]. To tackle uncertainties in determining HCV GT and ST, Sanger sequencing could be utilised to resolve indeterminate or discordant GTs or ST results produced by commercial assays [10, 11]. Despite the ability to provide definitive genotyping information most of the time, unfavourable features of Sanger sequencing including low throughput, time-consuming procedures and relatively high costs, pose a barrier to it becoming routinely adopted as a first-line genotyping method. With the advent of next-generation sequencing (NGS), limitations of probe-based genotyping assays and Sanger sequencing for HCV genotyping can be overcome. NGS provides a high-resolution means for direct sequence-based interrogation of the HCV genome. Moreover, NGS also allows concurrent profiling of RAVs where such value-added feature is highly relevant for the clinical management of HCV infection with appropriate use of DAAs.

In the present study, the Sentosa SQ HCV genotyping assay (hereinafter referred to as Vela NGS) (Vela Diagnostics, Singapore) which primarily interrogates the NS5B region of HCV GTs 1–6 by ion torrent-based NGS technology, was evaluated in comparison to the VERSANT HCV Genotype 2.0 Assay (hereinafter referred to as LiPA) (Siemens Healthineers, Erlangen, Germany). HCV indeterminate GTs previously reported in clinical samples by LiPA were resolved using Vela NGS assay with further confirmation by Sanger sequencing. Information on RAVs was also harnessed from deeply sequenced NS3, NS5A and NS5B regions in samples classified as HCV 1a and 1b using Vela NGS.

2. Study design

2.1 Clinical samples

This study was performed on residual sera or plasma from 222 clinical specimens previously received for routine genotyping using the VERSANT HCV Genotype 2.0 Line Probe Assay (Siemens Healthineers, Erlangen, Germany). All samples were stored at -80°C post-LiPA analysis and were only thawed prior to re-analysis by NGS and Sanger sequencing. All samples were de-identified for anonymisation purposes, and hence, the treatment histories remain unknown and cannot be traced. These were all residual samples, which would otherwise be discarded, and were used for the purposes of assay validation only. In such situations, ethics approval is not normally required, as all samples could not be linked back to the original patients after anonymisation.

2.2 NGS by Sentosa SQ HCV genotyping assay

In this study, NGS was performed using Sentosa SQ HCV Genotyping Assay (4 × 16) (Vela Diagnostics, Singapore) according to the manufacturer's instructions. The workflow started with automated extraction of total nucleic acids from 530 μL of sera or plasma using Sentosa SX Virus Total Nucleic Acid Plus II kit (Vela Diagnostics) on Sentosa SX101 (Vela Diagnostics). PCR amplification of the HCV NS3, NS5A and NS5B regions was performed on Veriti 96-Well Thermal Cycler (Applied Biosystems, CA, USA). In every individual run, a pooled library containing barcoded amplicons of 15 clinical samples and one system control, was prepared by Sentosa SX101. The pooled library was subject to sequencing template preparation and enrichment on Sentosa ST401 (Vela Diagnostics). Sequencing data generated by Sentosa SQ301 (Vela Diagnostics) was automatically channelled for primary and subsequent secondary analyses using Sentosa SQ Suite (Vela Diagnostics) and Sentosa SQ Reporter (Vela Diagnostics), respectively. Auto-generated quality control and pathology reports containing technical information, viral typing, and RAVs (available only for GTs 1a and 1b) results were manually reviewed, respectively.

2.3 VERSANT HCV Genotype 2.0 Line Probe Assay

Total nucleic acids were extracted from 200 μL sera or plasma using EZ1 Virus Mini Kit v2.0 (QIAGEN, Hilden, Germany) on Biorobot EZ1 (QIAGEN). Using VERSANT HCV Genotype 2.0 Line Probe Assay (LiPA) (Siemens Healthineers), a one-step reverse transcription-polymerase chain reaction (RT-PCR) amplifying the 5'UTR and core regions was performed on GeneAmp PCR System 9700 (Applied Biosystems). Reverse hybridisation, washing and colour development steps were performed on Autoblot 3000H (Fujirebio Europe, Gent, Belgium). For GT and ST determination, band patterns were manually scored by aligning the strips to an interpretation chart provided by the manufacturer.

2.4 Sanger sequencing

Sanger sequencing was performed on samples previously reported by LiPA as indeterminate genotype. A primary PCR amplification of a 454 bp fragment of the NS5B region was initially attempted using primers 5Bo8254 and 5Bo8707 [12]. In samples with PCR failure using the above-mentioned primers, a secondary PCR amplifying a 446 bp fragment of the 5'UTR/core regions was subsequently performed using primers UTR45 and Cor490 [12]. PCR products from the amplifiable gene segments were subjected to direct sequencing with BigDye Terminator v3.1 Cycle Sequencing kit (Applied Biosystems) using the respective PCR primers on a 3130XL Genetic Analyzer (Applied Biosystems).

2.5 Sequence analysis

Sequence analysis was performed by querying the nucleotide sequences obtained from Sanger sequencing in the Los Alamos hepatitis C sequence database [13]. For Vela NGS, assembled contigs were downloaded from the Sentosa SQ Reporter software. In samples with discordant results between LiPA and Vela NGS, NGS contigs were uploaded to the Los Alamos hepatitis C sequence database [13] to verify Vela NGS results.

3. Results

3.1 Concordance between results generated by the Vela NGS and Versant platforms at GT and ST levels

The Vela NGS results at both GT and ST levels were tabulated in **Table 1** for 170 clinical samples with GT and/or ST results from LiPA. Perfect (100%) concordance at HCV genotype level was achieved in GT 2 (N = 13), GT 3 (N = 55) and GT 5 (N = 7). For samples reported by LiPA as GT 1 (N = 40), 20% (N = 8) gave discrepant results when compared to Vela NGS. These samples had been previously classified by LiPA as either GT 1a with core inconclusive, GT 1b with 96.1% homology, GT 1b with core inconclusive, or GT 1b with core not available, due to their unconventional band patterns. There was no discrepancy between samples firmly reported as GT 1a and GT 1b by LiPA. In samples reported as GT 4 (N = 16) by LiPA, 43.8% (N = 7) were found to be GT 3 by Vela NGS. Two samples (5.1%) originally reported by LiPA as GT 3 were classified by Vela NGS as GT 6 samples.

At ST level, Vela NGS reclassified 1 sample previously assigned as HCV 1a with core inconclusive by LiPA as 1c. Two samples each reported as 4a/4c/4d and 4e by LiPA, respectively, were reclassified as 4n and 4o by Vela NGS. Another 29 GT 6 (ST c-l) samples reported by LiPA were reassigned by Vela NGS as 6e/6u (N = 1), 6j (N = 1), 6m (N = 9), and 6n (N = 18), respectively. One sample with LiPA 6m (77.9% homology) was reassigned as 6u by Vela NGS.

3.2 Verification of contig sequences generated by the Vela NGS in samples with discordant results

Of the 170 samples tested, there were 104 agreements at both GT and ST levels, 49 partial agreements at genotype but not the subtype levels, and 117 discordant results generated by LiPA and Vela NGS (**Table 1**). At GT level, the calculated Cohen's Kappa is 0.869 (95% confidence interval: 0.810–0.928), suggesting good strength of agreement between the two assays. The 66 NGS contig sequences of samples with partial agreement or discordant results were submitted to the online analysis in the Los Alamos hepatitis C sequence database. HCV GT and ST called by Vela NGS were verified in all 66 contigs.

3.3 Intra-run and inter-run reproducibility on GT and ST calling by Vela NGS

HCV genotyping and subtyping results were found to be reproducible for a panel of 5 samples with different HCV GT/ST including 1a, 1b, 2a, 3a and 3b tested in triplicates within a single run on the Vela NGS platform (**Figure 1a**). For inter-run reproducibility testing (**Figure 1b**), GT and ST results were consistently reported in another panel of 7 samples including 1a, 1b, 2b, 3a, 4d, 5a and 6n, which were repeatedly tested in three separate runs on different days. Details of viral load and median coverage of the targeted NS5B region are depicted in **Figure 1a** and **b**, respectively.

3.4 RAV analysis in GT 1 samples reported by the Vela NGS platform

In the current Vela NGS assay, a list of variants differing from the wild-type codons are detectable for HCV 1a and 1b. The 16 target codons in the NS3 gene are 36, 41, 43, 54, 55, 80, 109, 122, 132 (1a only), 138, 155, 156, 158, 168, 170 (1b only) and 175 (1b only). For NS5A, variants at nine codons including 28 (1a only), 30 (1a only), 31, 32, 54 (1b only), 58, 62 (1b only), 92 and 93, are detectable. Eight codons in the NS5B gene including 414, 419, 422, 423, 495, 499 (1b only), 554 and 559, are also covered in this assay.

Of 13 GT 1a samples (**Table 2**), five were found to carry at least one target variant in the NS3 gene. Notably, two samples carried the Q80K RAV. For NS5A, the M28A variant was detected in one sample in which NS3 Q80K was also present. None of the GT 1a samples was found to carry any of target variants in the NS5B gene.

Of 18 HCV 1b samples (**Table 2**), five were detected with at least one target variant in the NS3 gene. Twelve samples were identified with at least one target variant in the NS5A gene. For NS5B, the P495A and V499A variants were detected in one and eight samples, respectively. Notably, there were four samples detected with at least one target variant in each of the NS3, NS5A and NS5B genes.

3.5 Intra-run and inter-run reproducibility on variant calling and frequency

In intra-run reproducibility analysis, the Q80K variant was reproducibly detected in the NS3 gene of the GT 1a samples. Another two variants, namely Q54H

Table 1.
Comparison of GT and ST distribution in 170 samples tested by both LiPA and Vela NGS.

a In LiPA, the possibility of GT 6 (ST's 6 (ST's c-l) can not be excluded in HCV 1a or 1b with inconclusive or unevaluable core regions.
b LiPA bands 3, 4, 6, 1, 6 & 26
c Bands 13, 178, 24
d Bands 6, 7, 17, 18 & 24
e Bands 3, 4, 138, 24, 1 Bands 68, 24

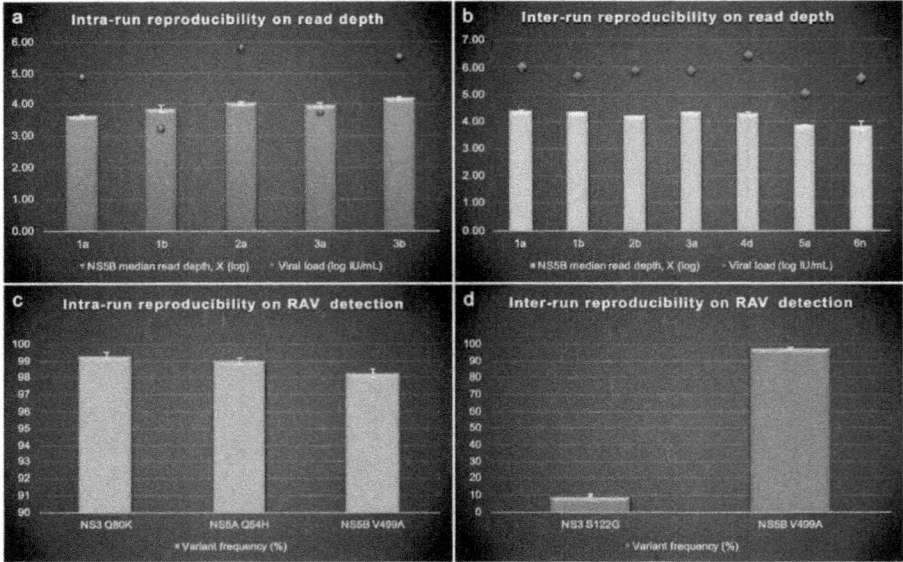

Figure 1.
Precision studies on the Vela NGS. (a) Intra-run and (b) inter-run reproducibility on median read depth were tested on 5 and 7 clinical specimens, respectively. For RAV analysis, variants were called with reproducible frequency (c) within a run (intra-run) and (d) between runs (inter-run).

No	ID	GT1 STs	RAVs (variant frequency)		
			NS3	NS5A	NS5B
1	R02-BC02	1a	S122G (99.21%), D168E (97.07%)	–	–
2	R02-BC03	1a	V55A (91.44%)	–	–
3	R02-BC04	1a	Q80K (25.63%)	M28V (99.47%)	–
4	R02-BC05	1a	Q80K (4.84%)	–	–
5	R13-BC13	1a	D168E (51.43%)	–	–
6	R01-BC02	1b	Q80K (55.29%) M175L (87.81%)	–	V499A (98.15%)
7	R01-BC03	1b	–	–	V499A (97.03%)
8	R01-BC04	1b	–	L31M (22.03%), Q54H (98.82%)	V499A (33.65%)
9	R01-BC05	1b	–	Q54H (99.11%), Y93H (99.73%)	–
10	R01-BC06	1b	Q80L (99.52%), S122G (9.99%)	Q54H (99.05%)	V499A (97.91%)
11	R01-BC07	1b	–	Q54H (98.76%), Y93H (99.61%)	–
12	R01-BC08	1b	–	Q54H (99.22%), Q62E (99.04%)	–
13	R01-BC09	1b	S122G (97.69%)	Q54H (99.21%), Q62E (51.64%)	P495A 8.83%
14	R01-BC11	1b	–	Y93H (99.24%)	–

No	ID	GT1 STs	RAVs (variant frequency)		
			NS3	NS5A	NS5B
15	R02-BC07	1b	–	Q54H (99.37%)	V499A 98.9%
16	R02-BC-11	1b	Q80R (92.29%)	Q62E (5.61%)	V499A 95.15%
17	R11-BC14	1b	M175L (99.97%)	Y93H (99.8%)	V499A 98.7%
18	R12-BC14	1b	–	Q54H (80.35%), Y93H (8.07%)	–
19	R12-BC15	1b	–	Q54H (98.82%), Q62R (99.79%)	–

In this study, RAVs with variant frequency less than 1% are not shown.

Table 2.
List of resistance-associated variants (RAVs) identified in GT 1a and 1b samples by Vela NGS.

No	LiPA results (bands)	Vela NGS	Sanger sequencing		Concordance at GT or ST level
			NS5B	5'UTR/core	
1	Indeterminate (3,6,16,24)	6n	Not amplified	6n	GT & ST
2	Indeterminate (3,6,16,24)	6n	Not amplified	6n	GT & ST
3	Indeterminate (3,6,16,24)	6n	Not amplified	6n	GT & ST
4	Indeterminate (6,7,24)	3b	3b	Not done	GT & ST
5	Indeterminate (6,7,24)	6m/6u	Not amplified	6e/6d	**GT only**
6	Indeterminate (6,7)	6u	6u/6n	Not done	GT & ST
7	Indeterminate (6,7)	6u	6m/6n	Not done	**GT only**
8	Indeterminate (6,7)	6u	6n/6a	Not done	**GT only**
9	Indeterminate (6)	6m/6l	6d/6e	Not done	**GT only**
10	Indeterminate (17,24)	3b	3b	Not done	GT & ST
11	Indeterminate (17,18,24)	3b	3b	Not done	GT & ST
12	Indeterminate (6,17,24)	3b	3b	Not done	GT & ST
13	Indeterminate (7,8,14,15,24)	3a	3a	Not done	GT & ST
14	Indeterminate (7,13,17,18)	3b	3b	Not done	GT & ST
15	Indeterminate (7,13,17,18,24)	3b	3b	Not done	GT & ST
16	Indeterminate (13,16,17,18,24)	3b	3b	Not done	GT & ST
17	Indeterminate (13,14,15,18,24)	3b	3b	Not done	GT & ST
18	Indeterminate (3,4,13,25)	1a	1a	Not done	GT & ST
19	Indeterminate (3,4,7,13,25)	1a	1a	Not done	GT & ST
20	Indeterminate (3,4,7,13,24)	6e	6e	Not done	GT & ST
21	Indeterminate (3,4,6,7,13,24)	6e	Not amplified	6e/6d	GT & ST
22	Indeterminate (5,9,21,24)	6a	Not amplified	6a	GT & ST
23	Indeterminate (5,6,9,17,18)	4a	Not amplified	4a	GT & ST
24	Indeterminate (5,9,10,13,14,15,24)	2a & 3a	Two mixed sequences	Not done	Likely mixed infections
25	Indeterminate (5,8,9,11)	2a	2a	Not done	GT & ST
26	Indeterminate (24)	3b	3b	Not done	GT & ST

No	LiPA results (bands)	Vela NGS	Sanger sequencing		Concordance at GT or ST level
			NS5B	5'UTR/core	
27	Indeterminate (24)	3b	3b	Not done	GT & ST
28	Indeterminate (4,5,9,16,21,24)	6a	6a	Not done	GT & ST
29	Indeterminate (4,9,21)	6a	Not amplified	6a	GT & ST
30	Indeterminate (3,4,6,13,17,18,24,26)	3b	3b	Not done	GT & ST
31	Indeterminate (6)	6n/6a	6d/6u	Not done	**GT only**
32	Indeterminate (3,4,13,25)	1a	1a	Not done	GT & ST
33	Indeterminate (6)	6u	6u	Not done	GT & ST
34	Indeterminate (13,16,24)	3b	3b	Not done	GT & ST
35	Indeterminate (7)	6u	Not amplified	6v/6l/6d/6k	**GT only**
36	Indeterminate (17,18,24)	3b	3b	Not done	GT & ST
37	Indeterminate (3,4,5,16,25)	1a	Not amplified	1a	GT & ST
38	Indeterminate (5,6,18,24)	3k	3k	Not done	GT & ST
39	Indeterminate (8,9,21,24)	6a	6a	Not done	GT & ST
40	Indeterminate (3,4,6,16,24)	6q	6q	Not done	GT & ST

PCR amplification for NS5B was first attempted in all 40 specimens. A secondary PCR amplifying 5'UTR/core regions were performed in samples with unsuccessful amplification of NS5B. Sanger sequencing was performed on PCR amplicon obtained.

Table 3.
Comparison of genotyping results produced by the Vela NGS and Sanger sequencing methods in 40 specimens with indeterminate genotypes by LiPA.

and V499A were also repeatedly identified in the NS5A and NS5B genes of the GT 1b sample, respectively. Variant frequencies of the three variants were highly reproducible within run (**Figure 1c**).

In the inter-run reproducibility study, NS3 S122G and NS5B V499A variants were tested. Variant frequencies of the two variants were found to be highly reproducible among the three separate runs (**Figure 1d**).

3.6 Vela NGS assigned HCV GT and ST to samples with indeterminate LiPA results

Forty specimens, which were previously reported as HCV indeterminate GT by LiPA, were subject to Vela NGS analysis. Sanger sequencing were successfully performed on NS5b (N = 30) or 5'UTR/core (N = 10) regions in 40 samples (**Table 3**). Of the 40 samples with Sanger sequencing results, Vela NGS results were confirmed at GT level in 39 samples (97.5%). In a sample with LiPA complex band patterns (5, 9, 10, 13, 14, 15 & 24), a mixed genotypes of GT 2a and GT 3a were assigned by Vela NGS. Sanger sequencing on NS5B showed overlapping nucleotide base calls in the overall sequences, in which putative mixed infection with two different HCV GTs was likely inferred.

4. Discussion

The application of NGS assays to analyse quasispecies HCV genomes has been increasing in recent years. Several laboratory-developed NGS assays had been previously described in the literature for phylogenetic studies [14], outbreak investigation [15, 16], characterisation of HCV full genome [17, 18] and identification of HCV GT and ST in clinical samples [19, 20]. However, there are fewer reports of adoption of NGS assays in routine HCV genotyping. In 2016, Vela NGS became available as a CE-IVD certified commercial kit for diagnostic use in the clinical laboratories. In this study, we report the performance characteristics of Vela NGS in comparison to the widely used LiPA assay for HCV genotyping.

The performance of Vela NGS in determining the HCV GT and ST in the clinical specimens had been discussed in several previous studies [21–23]. Perfect agreement at GT level was observed between Vela NGS and LiPA in a study by Manee et al. [21]. Samples with unclear ST results in GTs 2, 3, 4 and 6 reported by LiPA were each assigned with a specific subtype after subject to Vela NGS analysis. Dirani et al. [22] also performed a direct comparison of GT and ST calling between Vela NGS and LiPA for samples from patients infected with HCV GTs including GT 1, 2, 3 and 4, and found a high concordance (>99%) at GT level between the two tests. Vela NGS was also found to have better performance in assigning HCV STs among the four GTs when compared to LiPA [22]. In another study by Rodriguez et al. [23], Vela NGS achieved high concordance rates with Sanger sequencing in assigning GTs 1 to 6, 1a and 1b STs, and other STs for GTs 4, 5 and 6. Discrepant calls at ST level was mainly found among HCV GTs 1 and 2 between Vela NGS and Sanger sequencing; the latter was used as the reference method to sequence the 286 bp segment of NS5B for which phylogenetic analysis was performed.

In the present study, discrepancy in results was mainly observed in samples with LiPA GT 1b with incomplete or missing bands at the core region. In this particular result group, GT 6 with different STs were assigned by Vela NGS. This observation was not unexpected as it has been specified in the LiPA interpretation chart that GT 6 (STs c-1) cannot be differentiated from ST 1a and 1b without additional information from the core region sequence. Among LiPA GT 4 samples, all ST 4h were reassigned as GT 3 by Vela NGS. Some geographical regions, for example, Southeast Asia, where GT 6 is highly prevalent [24], could thus be impacted more by this misclassification with the use of LiPA method.

In contrast to LiPA which utilises primarily the 5'UTR in GTs 1-6 and core regions for the discrimination of GT 6 STs c-l from 1a and 1b, Vela NGS targets the non-structural genes implicated in both accurate genotyping/subtyping and resistance to DAAs. The LiPA is known to be poor at detecting and identifying recombinant forms of HCV [25]. Due to the assay design of Vela NGS, this may also pose a problem for this platform, despite the application of NGS technology. The HCV recombinant forms can be accurately detected via sequencing of recombination breakpoint junctions or the whole HCV genome [26]. For example, in our study, one previously LiPA-indeterminate sample was reported by the Vela NGS to have mixed HCV infections with HCV 2a and 3a. This NGS finding was confirmed by Sanger sequencing in which overlapping Sanger electropherograms were observed for NS5B.

The Vela NGS offers information on RAVs in HCV 1a or 1b positive samples, where such profiling will be useful when prescribing DAA regimes, and detecting of baseline or emerging RAVs. Targeted assays had been previously developed to identify a specific RAV [27, 28]. RAVs which are found at levels with at least 15% variant frequency, at baseline, are known to confer resistance to certain DAAs [29], and therefore may impact on the effectiveness of DAA treatment [30]. Vela NGS targets relevant RAVs in three non-structural gene segments (NS3, NS5A and NS5B) of HCV 1a and 1b, and although the RAV profiling is comprehensive but not exhaustive due to the assay design, any baseline RAVs present in any of these DAA target genes, can affect the therapeutic effectiveness [31]. In our study, four HCV 1b samples were found to harbour variants in all three NS3, NS5A and NS5B genes concurrently.

5. Conclusions

In conclusion, the genotyping results of the Vela NGS were found to be highly concordant with those of the LiPA method. Vela NGS refined the ST assignment in GT 6 and resolved previously indeterminate GTs reported by LiPA. Technically, the HCV Vela NGS was found to have consistent intra- and inter-run reproducibility in terms of GT and ST calling and RAVs identification. Detection of infections with multiple HCV GTs or STs is feasible by Vela NGS. Due to the assay design which relies on investigating the HCV sub-genomic regions, HCV recombinant strains may still be potentially missed. Deep sequencing allows sensitive identification of RAVs in the GT1a and 1b NS3, NS5A and NS5B regions, but the list of target RAVs is not exhaustive. We would also suggest the RAVs detection spectrum should be extended to cover GTs other than HCV 1a and 1b, namely GTs 2-6.

Acknowledgements

We thank Cui-Wen Chua, Mui-Joo Khoo and Lily Chiu of the Department of Laboratory Medicine at the National University Hospital, Singapore, for their technical assistance in performing the NGS and LiPA analysis. We also thank Vela Diagnostics Singapore for funding the NGS reagents in this study.

Conflict of interest

The authors have no conflict of interest to declare.

Author details

Kok-Siong Poon[1], Julian Wei-Tze Tang[2] and Evelyn Siew-Chuan Koay[1,3]*

1 Department of Laboratory Medicine, National University Hospital, Singapore

2 University Hospitals of Leicester NHS, Leicester, United Kingdom

3 Department of Pathology, Yong Loo Lin School of Medicine, National University of Singapore, Singapore

*Address all correspondence to: evelyn_koay@nuhs.edu.sg

IntechOpen

References

[1] Murphy DG, Sablon E, Chamberland J, Fournier E, Dandavino R, et al. Hepatitis C virus genotype 7, a new genotype originating from central Africa. Journal of Clinical Microbiology. 2015;**53**:967-972

[2] Ghany MG, Strader DB, Thomas DL, Seeff LB. Diagnosis, management, and treatment of hepatitis C: An update. Hepatology. 2009;**49**:1335-1374

[3] ASLD-IDSA HCV Guidance Panel. Hepatitis C guidance 2018 update: AASLD-IDSA recommendations for testing, managing, and treating hepatitis C virus infection. Clinical Infectious Diseases. 2018

[4] Germer JJ, Majewski DW, Rosser M, Thompson A, Mitchell PS, et al. Evaluation of the TRUGENE HCV 5'NC genotyping kit with the new GeneLibrarian module 312 for genotyping of hepatitis C virus from clinical specimens. Journal of Clinical Microbiology. 2003;**41**:4855-4857

[5] Verbeeck J, Stanley MJ, Shieh J, Celis L, Huyck E, et al. Evaluation of Versant hepatitis C virus genotype assay (LiPA) 2.0. Journal of Clinical Microbiology. 2008;**46**:1901-1906

[6] González V, Gomes-Fernandes M, Bascuñana E, Casanovas S, Saludes V, et al. Accuracy of a commercially available assay for HCV genotyping and subtyping in the clinical practice. Journal of Clinical Virology. 2013;**58**:249-253

[7] Némoz B, Roger L, Leroy V, Poveda JD, Morand P, et al. Evaluation of the cobas® GT hepatitis C virus genotyping assay in G1-6 viruses including low viral loads and LiPA failures. PLoS One. 2018;**13**:e0194396

[8] Fernández-Caballero JA, Alvarez M, Chueca N, Pérez AB, García F. The cobas® HCV GT is a new tool that accurately identifies Hepatitis C virus genotypes for clinical practice. PLoS One. 2017;**12**:e0175564

[9] Benedet M, Adachi D, Wong A, Wong S, Pabbaraju K, Tellier R, et al. The need for a sequencing-based assay to supplement the Abbott m2000 RealTime HCV Genotype II assay: A 1 year analysis. Journal of Clinical Virology. 2014;**60**:301-304

[10] Larrat S, Poveda JD, Coudret C, Fusillier K, Magnat N, et al. Sequencing assays for failed genotyping with the versant hepatitis C virus genotype assay (LiPA), version 2.0. Journal of Clinical Microbiology. 2013;**51**:2815-2821

[11] Chueca N, Rivadulla I, Lovatti R, Reina G, Blanco A, et al. Using NS5B sequencing for hepatitis C virus genotyping reveals discordances with commercial platforms. PLoS One. 2016;**11**:e0153754

[12] Quer J, Gregori J, Rodríguez-Frias F, Buti M, Madejon A, et al. High-resolution hepatitis C virus subtyping using NS5B deep sequencing and phylogeny, an alternative to current methods. Journal of Clinical Microbiology. 2015;**53**:219-226

[13] Kuiken C, Yusim K, Boykin L, Richardson R. The Los Alamos hepatitis C sequence database. Bioinformatics. 2005;**1**:379-384

[14] Gonçalves Rossi LM, Escobar-Gutierrez A, Rahal P. Multiregion deep sequencing of hepatitis C virus: An improved approach for genetic relatedness studies. Infection, Genetics and Evolution. 2016;**38**:138-145

[15] Escobar-Gutiérrez A, Vazquez-Pichardo M, Cruz-Rivera M, Rivera-Osorio P, Carpio-Pedroza JC, et al. Identification of hepatitis C virus

transmission using a next-generation sequencing approach. Journal of Clinical Microbiology. 2012;**50**:1461-1463

[16] Caraballo Cortes K, Rosińska M, Janiak M, Stępień M, Zagordi O, et al. Next-generation sequencing analysis of a cluster of hepatitis C virus infections in a haematology and oncology center. PLoS One. 2018;**13**:e0194816

[17] Salmona M, Caporossi A, Simmonds P, Thélu MA, Fusillier K, et al. First next-generation sequencing full-genome characterization of a hepatitis C virus genotype 7 divergent subtype. Clinical Microbiology and Infection. 2016;**22**:e1-e947

[18] Thomson E, Ip CL, Badhan A, Christiansen MT, Adamson W, et al. Comparison of next-generation sequencing technologies for comprehensive assessment of full-length hepatitis C viral genomes. Journal of Clinical Microbiology. 2016;**54**:2470-2484

[19] Pedersen MS, Fahnøe U, Hansen TA, Pedersen AG, Jenssen H, et al. A near full-length open reading frame next generation sequencing assay for genotyping and identification of resistance-associated variants in hepatitis C virus. Journal of Clinical Virology. 2018;**195**:49-56

[20] Del Campo JA, Parra-Sánchez M, Figueruela B, García-Rey S, Quer J, et al. Hepatitis C virus deep sequencing for sub-genotype identification in mixed infections: A real-life experience. International Journal of Infectious Diseases. 2018;**67**:114-117

[21] Manee N, Thongbaiphet N, Pasomsub E, Chantratita W. Clinical evaluation of a newly developed automated massively parallel sequencing assay for hepatitis C virus genotyping and detection of resistance-association variants Comparison with a line probe assay. Journal of Virological Methods. 2017;**249**:31-37

[22] Dirani G, Paesini E, Mascetra E, Farabegoli P, Dalmo B, et al. A novel next generation sequencing assay as an alternative to currently available methods for hepatitis C virus genotyping. Journal of Virological Methods. 2018;**251**:88-91

[23] Rodriguez C, Soulier A, Demontant V, Poiteau L, Mercier-Darty M, et al. A novel standardized deep sequencing-based assay for hepatitis C virus genotype determination. Scientific Reports. 2018;**8**:4180

[24] Bunchorntavakul C, Chavalitdhamrong D, Tanwandee T. Hepatitis C genotype 6: A concise review and response-guided therapy proposal. World Journal of Hepatology. 2013;**5**:496-504

[25] Schuermans W, Orlent H, Desombere I, Descheemaeker P, Van Vlierberghe H, et al. Heads or tails: Genotyping of hepatitis C virus concerning the 2k/1b circulating recombinant form. International Journal of Molecular Sciences. 2016;**17**

[26] Iles JC, Njouom R, Foupouapouognigni Y, Bonsall D, Bowden R, et al. Characterization of hepatitis c virus recombination in Cameroon by use of nonspecific next-generation sequencing. Journal of Clinical Microbiology. 2015;**53**:3155-3164

[27] Chui CK, Dong WW, Joy JB, Poon AF, Dong WY, et al. Development and validation of two screening assays for the hepatitis C virus NS3 Q80K polymorphism associated with reduced response to combination treatment regimens containing simeprevir. Journal of Clinical Microbiology. 2015;**53**:2942-2950

[28] Vicenti I, Falasca F, Sticchi L, Bruzzone B, Turriziani O, et al. Evaluation of a commercial real-time PCR kit for the detection of the Q80K

polymorphism in plasma from HCV genotype 1a infected patients. Journal of Clinical Virology. 2016;**76**:20-23

[29] Pawlotsky JM. Hepatitis C virus resistance to direct-acting antiviral drugs in interferon-free regimens. Gastroenterology. 2016;**151**:70-86

[30] Yoshida K, Hai TA, Teranishi Y, Kozuka R, et al. Long-term follow-up of resistance-associated substitutions in hepatitis C virus in patients in which direct acting antiviral-based therapy failed. International Journal of Molecular Sciences. 2017;**18**

[31] Mawatari S, Oda K, Tabu K, Ijuin S, Kumagai K. New resistance-associated substitutions and failure of dual oral therapy with daclatasvir and asunaprevir. Journal of Gastroenterology. 2017;**52**:855-867